AF713218

The Death Care Industry and Urban Gun Violence

Melvin Delgado

The Death Care Industry and Urban Gun Violence

Helping Profession Strategies for Engagement and Support

Springer

Melvin Delgado
School of Social Work
Boston University
Boston, MA, USA

ISBN 978-3-031-95681-2 ISBN 978-3-031-95682-9 (eBook)
https://doi.org/10.1007/978-3-031-95682-9

© The Editor(s) (if applicable) and The Author(s), under exclusive license to Springer Nature Switzerland AG 2025

This work is subject to copyright. All rights are solely and exclusively licensed by the Publisher, whether the whole or part of the material is concerned, specifically the rights of translation, reprinting, reuse of illustrations, recitation, broadcasting, reproduction on microfilms or in any other physical way, and transmission or information storage and retrieval, electronic adaptation, computer software, or by similar or dissimilar methodology now known or hereafter developed.
The use of general descriptive names, registered names, trademarks, service marks, etc. in this publication does not imply, even in the absence of a specific statement, that such names are exempt from the relevant protective laws and regulations and therefore free for general use.
The publisher, the authors and the editors are safe to assume that the advice and information in this book are believed to be true and accurate at the date of publication. Neither the publisher nor the authors or the editors give a warranty, expressed or implied, with respect to the material contained herein or for any errors or omissions that may have been made. The publisher remains neutral with regard to jurisdictional claims in published maps and institutional affiliations.

This Springer imprint is published by the registered company Springer Nature Switzerland AG
The registered company address is: Gewerbestrasse 11, 6330 Cham, Switzerland

If disposing of this product, please recycle the paper.

This book is dedicated to those on the front lines fighting against gun violence!

Contents

About the Author

Melvin Delgado, PhD, is emeritus professor of social work at Boston University School of Social Work. Delgado has devoted his career to research and scholarship focused on urban issues and strategies. The subject of gun violence, particularly when centered on this nation's urban centers and among residents of color, has been the focus of his scholarly attention over the past 3 years. Delgado has published approximately 40 books on a range of urban topics including community practice, gun violence, businesses, research, vacant gardens, and Latinos.

Part I
Setting the Foundation

Chapter 1
Introduction to the Journey

Introduction

Setting a book's foundation introduces key goals that any "good" foundation seeks to achieve, whether we are building a house, filming a movie, playing any game, or helping our children navigate life's trials and tribulations. A book on gun violence and the death care sector brings additional challenges that cannot be ignored due to the topic's importance, complexity, and emotionality. This chapter provides parameters on a subject that is expanding into new arenas, with the death care sector the latest venture, bringing a host of challenges for victims, their families, neighborhoods, and the nation. The rewards of venturing into this new terrain and using different lens far outweigh the challenges, with the nation better by broadening the boundary and context of what constitutes urban community practice.

A book's first chapter either engages or loses readers. It is my most anticipated chapter from a reader's standpoint. I select a book to read based on the title, author (reputation), and the brief description typically provided to capture a reader's attention. In this case, a "good" introductory chapter has three important goals: (1) engaging readers in the importance of the journey and providing a roadmap for how this book will unfold; (2) explaining why death care services are significant for the nation, its urban communities of color, and helping professions; and (3) helping readers appreciate why urban gun violence is worthy of an entire book being devoted to this sector and topic. Even when this book is focused in this manner, readers will have only scratched the proverbial surface. Hopefully, this book spurs further reading on this subject and a willingness to take a road less traveled, per Robert Frost's poem.

My hope is that readers well versed on urban gun violence experience a "new" arena or contextual grounding, expanding their vision and knowledge, and bringing a spotlight that engenders innovative approaches to this national public health problem. Successfully addressing gun violence requires initiatives that address

© The Author(s), under exclusive license to Springer Nature Switzerland AG 2025

M. Delgado, *The Death Care Industry and Urban Gun Violence*,
https://doi.org/10.1007/978-3-031-95682-9_1

disenfranchised (grief unacknowledged by society) communities and the ills that compromise hope for a better future.

This book expands conventional views on the gun violence field, bringing together occasion, place, and space to a tragic event, allowing grounding of statistics and personal stories to be viewed, understood, and appropriately addressed. Urban practice draws on a plethora of theoretical groundings to assess, plan, and implement interventions. This "eclectic" view facilitates local circumstances shaping assessment, planning, and implementing interventions.

For readers well versed on gun violence, much of this material will serve as a "refresher." Those new to this subject will have a foundation to view this venture into the death care sector, which is multi-faceted and community-centered. This stance offers a potential route to take in practice and research in reaching urban communities of color dealing with gun-related deaths, including the community trauma it brings. This stance brings excitement and trepidation at the same time. That is code for an adventurous journey with getting to the destination being as much "fun" as being there. Mind you, this is not to say that there will be no bumps in the road.

All nations face immense challenges to their wellbeing and future. Some challenges relate to their geography, such as places where earthquakes or tsunamis are prone to occur bringing unprecedented injuries and deaths, as well as unpredictability. Famine is another challenge for some nations, with a slow death waiting to happen, with all of the miseries that brings for multiple generations. Some nations are engaged in **civil or war against aggressors**, which speaks to daily and severe pain of various types. Yet other nations face regular insurrections culminating in countless deaths and accompanying misery, bringing a history of instability in national leadership with corresponding ills.

There is no disputing that the United States, too, is facing challenges, ranging from internal threats to democracy to navigating daily life in this nation's most socially and economically challenged urban communities, with gun violence one of many challenges (Buggs, 2022; Buggs et al., 2023; Egodage, 2024; McMillan et al., 2024). Violence's manifestations have shaped this country's existence from its origins to the present-day, with guns increasingly playing an instrumental role in perpetrating this social problem in the modern day (See, 2018).

Gun deaths are a significant public health problem (Crandall et al., 2021; Hawkins, 2024). There is no disputing this conclusion. While we engage in intense debates about the freedom to own guns, tens of thousands every year fall victim to this problem. On June 24, 2024, the U.S. Surgeon General declared gun violence a national public health crisis, responsible for almost 40,000 deaths annually, or over 3000 per month or 100 per day; this calls for attention to initiatives worthy of such numbers, similar to those created to reduce smoking and motor vehicle crashes (Seitz, 2024). Those campaigns, unfortunately, took decades to unfold! Further, the courts are inclined to play a significant role in increasing gun availability, too.

One has only to look at D.C., the nation's capital, to see it as a symbol ("*Shining City on the Hill*") to the rest of the world. Washington D.C., nevertheless, has a gun violence problem that threatens its full-time residents and is symbolic of the challenge facing the nation (Hermann, 2023). We also have Washington, D.C. with politics, the nation's seat of power, and corresponding monuments to the dead. Within this highly marketed image, we have an invisible reality to the outside world that consists of pain and suffering caused by guns (Davies, 2024).

How many gun-related funerals are too many for a 14-year-old? Rashad, a resident of Washington, D.C., for example, has attended five services but it bears noting that the number could have been much higher because he missed several due to an inability to get rides or he simply did not have the stomach to attend others. No one of any age, let alone someone in their early teens, should have this experience with violent deaths. If this can happen in a nation's capital, nowhere or no one is immune from this violence and the corresponding misery it brings personally and collectively, including the seemingly permanent stain of blood on neighborhood streets.

There are numerous reasons why our nation has an international reputation for being a violent country, with concerns about gun violence on international travel advisories for visitors to the United States. There is little disputing that gun violence permeates this country, with no day going by without multiple gun injuries and deaths being reported by the local and national media. This brings profound emotional, physical, social, and economic consequences for victims, their families, neighborhoods, and the nation. Gun violence permeates the air that we breathe, literally and figuratively. In some communities, no place or occasion is safe from this violence, including its last rites ceremonies at funeral homes, cemeteries, and houses of worship.

Nationally, it was estimated that by the end of 2023, one in seven (14.3%) Americans lived within a quarter mile of a fatal gun shooting, expanding the conventional boundaries associated with this violence from one in nine (11.1%) prior to the COVID-19 epidemic (Karlamangia, 2024). This increase in deaths is largely due to greater gun availability, substance use/abuse, and gang activity, including police pulling back in response to local crime.

The scope of gun availability is arduous to grasp for the general public. However, one perspective helps (Everytown Research & Policy, 2023). In 2022, estimates had almost 78,000 licensed gun dealers in the United States. This is a greater number than all of this nation's McDonald's, Burger King's, Subway's, and Wendy's establishments combined; or, another perspective, has gun dealers representing twice the number of U.S. post offices!

There are multiple U.S. cities known nationally and internationally for gun violence. Philadelphia, for example, a city receiving considerable attention in this book, had one block consisting of 167 residents experiencing 64 killings, up from 24 in 2019, an increase of 266% (Murray et al., 2024). This number of gun deaths gives new meaning to "hot spots," making them more of a raging inferno than a hot spot! Gun violence is not evenly distributed throughout a community, displaying a propensity to occur within select spaces and places (Dong et al., 2024), with particularly high numbers of gun violence referred to as "hot spots," which will be discussed throughout this book.

Hot spots (excessive gun violence) is a concept with saliency among criminologists, but also in designating buildings and certain street corners, for example. Hot spots are not only concentrated in select spaces and places, but the gun violence perpetrated is also being done by a small group in a concentrated geographical area. That fact has not changed much over the past few decades since the concept initially gained saliency among criminologists. Boschan and Roman's (2024) study of hot spots in South Philadelphia highlighted the need for a classification system to designate areas on gun violence—new, consecutive, intensify, and persistent. Hot spot strategies have been found to be effective, as in the case of Dallas, when limited in geographical scope and time period (Smith et al., 2024).

No community can sustain a dramatic and sustained increase in gun violence over a period of years and decades and remain viable over time without suffering disastrous consequences. The same can be said for the nation. In the discussion on community trauma in Chap. 4, readers will see that one does not have to be a direct victim or related to one to experience the deleterious emotional and physical consequences of this violence, compounding other social problems facing these communities.

Black-Americans and Latinos have been disproportionately victims of this violence, and so have their families, social networks, communities, and key institutions. We cannot develop a comprehensive contextual understanding of racial disparities without taking gun violence into account as significant in shaping their manifestations (Hureau, 2022). The inability to stop this violence hampers our ability to develop effective and highly targeted interventions. Academics and healthcare providers will no doubt agree with this conclusion.

Threats to Black and Brown communities have a long history in this country, with guns the latest evolution and often without regard for who pays the ultimate price with their lives and how it compromises families and a neighborhood's existence. These communities and racial/ethnic groups, often primarily males, endure most of the direct consequences of this violence, including trauma (physical and emotional), which often goes unmentioned by media outlets (Armstrong & Carlson, 2019; Beard et al., 2023; Delgado, 2022; Henry et al., 2024). Male victims, in turn, can leave behind families, including very young children who will grow up without their biological father, increasing the chances that they, too, will face extreme hardships before they potentially face similar life-ending fates as their fathers (Hitchens, 2022).

Their remaining partners will bear the onus of raising children and attempting to keep them physically and emotionally safe in violent surroundings. Neighborhoods with exceedingly high gun violence rates take on the semblance of a community under war siege, with danger zones (hot spots) to be eschewed at all costs. They cannot "bullet-proof" their children, pardon the pun, as argued over 30 years ago (Richters & Martinez, 1993)! On the contrary, if they face the misfortunate of being shot, the injuries caused will likely have even more severe consequences to the body if they live to tell their stories to the next generation (Shorr, 2017). Therefore, joining the ranks of those with severe disabilities (physical and emotional) serves as constant reminders of the consequences of gun violence, compromising their remaining years.

The term “children born of war” (Frisso, 2024) is probably familiar to many readers, with their distressing visual images and severe consequences embedded in our minds, and futures severely compromised. This concept captures a series of conditions and challenges of growing up with a range of personal and environmental challenges, to put it mildly, that makes achieving adulthood difficult to imagine. This concept has not been applied to the United States, to the best of my knowledge, because there are communities that would qualify for this designation. Is this hyperbole? I do not think so.

Children of color in marginalized and violent communities, too, can be considered children born of war, with many of the same negative outcome circumstances we attribute to their counterparts in foreign countries under siege, but this is happening in our communities; this violence compromises key developmental stages, increasing the odds that they will be relegated to life’s margins. This war can be internally driven or in the case of police brutality, externally driven, compounding life in these neighborhoods. Yet, again, it can be both, with no demilitarized zones (DNZ) to provide temporary safety.

Our knowledge base is increasing on multiple gun violence dimensions, bringing hope for this field. Nevertheless, there is much to learn and do. We, for example, know relatively little of the needs and long-term ramifications of what happens to relatives who have experienced multiple family member killings and the toll this takes on them and their social network (Hitchens, 2023).

Longitudinal research is in short supply, limiting our understanding of gun violence to the immediate time period, which is a narrow view of this violence’s impact (Carter et al., 2021; Huesmann et al., 2021). Childhood trauma exposure and gun violence, for example, although requiring more extensive research, shows promising results in helping us better understand between this relationship (Wamser-Nanney et al., 2019). Understanding how developmental stages are influenced over a lifetime for young victims of gun violence, directly and indirectly in the case of those losing a parent or sibling, remains to be undertaken. The long-term social, economic, physical, and social consequences of gun violence is “scant” (Fahimi et al., 2016; Ganpo-Nkwenkwa et al., 2023; Orlas et al., 2021; Ranney et al., 2019).

Further, we think of gun deaths from an individualistic perspective with a stoplight on the direct victim and their demographic characteristics (race/ethnicity, age, and gender) standing out in media coverage, which is generally referred to as “episodic crime reporting” (Boncy, 2024), This can be expected in a highly individualistic nation. Nevertheless, what happens to families with multiple gun deaths? Surely, the ramifications will unfold in a more intense and long-lasting manner, as discussed in Chap. 4 on community trauma. Further, we know very little about those in the death care sector, particularly when children are victims, regardless of their ages. All deaths are never equal, although each death is significant, bringing its share of pain and sorrow. Just ask the parent(s) of a dead child! Finally, those working in the media doing the reporting of murders and injuries, too, suffer traumatic consequences (Cherry, 2023).

These deaths make those in the death care sector co-victims with all of the emotional consequences attached to this status. Gun violence statistics do not capture these injuries. This calls for additional research and development of comprehensive trauma- and grief-informed interventions that go beyond immediate family members and include providers, typical and untypical, as in the case of the death care sector and community trauma. Of course, readers can argue that the entire nation suffers from gun violence by creating fears of public spaces and places (Delgado, 2024), with no place or space free from this violence.

Gun Violence and the American Way

Although this book focuses on urban centers, it would be irresponsible to ignore that most gun violence between 2014 and 2023 occurred outside large cities, which get the major portion of publicity. The south's rural, small, and large towns had higher levels of gun violence than any other region of the country. Small cities and towns with populations under one million people have not escaped this violence. More specifically, 13 of the 20 towns and cities accounted for the highest rates of shootings can be found in the south, such as Selma, Alabama. Selma, for example, had the negative distinction of possessing a per capita shooting rate higher than Chicago (Pierce et al., 2024). Other examples have Clarksdale, Mississippi; Selma, Alabama; and Laurinburg, North Carolina, having higher gun victims on a per capita basis than Chicago, Illinois; Philadelphia, Pennsylvania; and Washington, D.C. Another perspective, over the past 9 years, has the rate of Black gunshot victims in places like Alabama and Mississippi being six times higher than in New York, New York or Los Angeles, California (Gore, 2024).

The saying that "*Gun violence is as American as Apple Pie*" requires us to pause and briefly ground the extent of gun ownership to better appreciate and understand the present-day situation involving this form of violence. The U.S. civilian population represents 5% of the world's population but owns almost half (46%) of all civilian guns (Gilligan, 2023). This arsenal makes gun access relatively easy, even when one is a resident of a state with high gun control laws. How did this country get to this point needs to be raised to appreciate the formidable challenges we face in addressing gun violence from a public health standpoint (Yamane, 2023):

> Before there was a gun industry, there were guns in the US. When the first colonists arrived at what would be called Jamestown in 1607 and Plymouth Rock in 1620, they had guns at the ready. Firearms continued to be commonly owned (by those who could legally do so) in the run-up to the colonists' Declaration of Independence from the British Crown and the nation's Constitutional founding. One reliable estimate of ownership rates in early America found firearms in 50 to 73 percent of male estates and even 6 to 38 percent of female estates. These rates compare favorably to other everyday items listed like swords or edged weapons (14% of estate inventories), Bibles (25%), or cash (30%). (p. 2)

We cannot separate guns from U.S. history, helping us better understand present-day gun violence and the challenges associated with gun control. Yet, there is something fundamentally different about gun ownership in the present-day because of the ready availability of these weapons to impose our will and our propensity to use them to settle disputes.

The emergence of assault weapons, it is necessary to uplift, introduces a lethality unprecedented in American history and the urban scene, and the cause of much of the misery covered in this book, including compromising last rite rituals with deep social and cultural roots. Assault weapons and large capacity magazines ("weapons of war") facilitate mass shootings transpiring within a relatively few seconds (Abbasi, 2020; Cook & Donohue, 2022). These are high precision weapons, causing widespread killing and hurting of bystanders. One study found that the probabilities of someone injured dying from being shot increases by 44% without regard to the type of weapon.

The professional literature is replete with examples of risk factors. Readers, as a result, are well-versed with the concept of risk factors across a wide terrain. Living in a high gun violence community is a risk factor regardless of resident socio-characteristics. When risk factors are applied to Black-American communities, for example, they are almost 14 times at greater risk to die by gun homicide than their White, non-Latino counterparts (Gillum et al., 2024).

The following overview illustrates what Black-American adults are facing: 71% of adults know or care for someone that has experienced gun violence in their lifetimes; 31% know or care about someone who was shot and wounded; one in three know or care about someone who was killed with a gun, with 57% of survivors experiencing trauma from the incident (Imes, 2024). Gun murders are this country's second leading cause of death for victims 15–19 years old from 2018 to 2021 (Puppala et al., 2024), behind unintentional injuries. These statistics are staggering when contemplating how lives are forever altered for their loved ones.

A semi-automatic weapon doubles the number of deaths, and not to mention the severity of injuries for survivors, illustrating this weapon's power to cause unimaginable destruction to the human body (Brigham, 2023). Survivor lives are forever changed and are destined to live with unimaginable injuries, compromising their lives and those of their immediate social network (Delgado, 2022).

The fate of corpses in mass violence has only recently drawn scholarly interests because of how they require special attention; they extract an immense psychic tax on the death care sector due to the nature and extensiveness of the damages to the body that they cause (Anstett et al., 2023). This interest has much to do with the destruction caused by semi-automatic weapons or the use of bump-stocks and the ability of shooters to cause wide destruction in a relatively short period of time, as per the Las Vegas October 1, 2017 mass shooting that left 61 dead and 413 wounded, with an additional 867 injured in the stampede that followed; an estimated 1000 rounds were fired.

How big is the U.S.'s gun violence problem? Let me further count the ways that gun ownership is unprecedented and difficult to grasp even visually unless you have personally experienced it in one form or another. It is best viewed at the micro, mezzo, and macro levels. National estimates have guns outnumbering residents by at least 50 million more (Webster, 2024), with 29% of owners with over five guns each! This arsenal of weapons symbolizes a menacing dark cloud on the horizon ready to bring down a storm of misery, death, and destruction. The question is not whether but when, as in now! It is definitely raining heavily now, and it is just a question of when the intensity gets fully manifested, with the pending doom following.

It is understandable why we as a society emphasize the consequences gun violence, including corresponding deaths, and on occasions injuries of various severities that will forever haunt victims because of their high visibility, as well as invisibility in the cause of emotional trauma. Infertility (abdominopelvic injuries), for instance, is another form of a life not lived and a hidden trauma that goes unrecorded with long-term demographic ramifications for communities and society (Adeleye et al., 2022). Ralph's (2014) breakthrough book *Renegade Dreams: Living through Injury in Gangland Chicago* highlights how physical injuries alter the life of gun victims and their loved ones, a group overlooked in the rush to document deaths while ignoring injuries.

The popularity of high-powered assault weapons meant for military war use to maximize destruction, as touched on earlier, further compounds the prevalence of weapons because of the destruction to the body that they cause and the ease in which is done (Menezes et al., 2023). Urban centers and events lend themselves to large crowds, resulting in mass casualties and injuries, irrespective of who is the target. Young children and older adults, including people with mobility impairments, are easy targets.

Gun violence complicates healing for survivors and burial practices for those who do not. Burials do not mean there will be everlasting peace for their families and neighborhoods. The sense that "it is never over" will haunt families of murdered victims, particularly when the perpetrators are not brought to justice. That sense of inevitable doom may be very hard to comprehend and indicative of how gun violence is an act that can cross generations for many families, leaving constant reminders for neighborhoods to witness.

Not surprisingly, there are countless reasons why gun violence has been designated a national public health epidemic and subject of increasing popular and scholarly attention (Fontanarosa & Bibbins-Domingo, 2022; Mueller et al., 2023; Sanchez et al., 2020). Popular media, too, has joined this coverage. Thus, practitioners, academics, including communities, face prodigious challenges in how best to prevent and treat gun victims, immediate and extended, of this violence, with subgroups such as youth and young adults standing out as targets.

"Shooting galleries" is a concept that historically captured urban spaces devoted to heroin injection, bringing their share of deaths due to overdoses. Now, I consider shooting galleries to symbolize spaces associated with misery and where multiple gun shootings transpire over a period of time. These shootings are increasingly, geographically clustered into "hot spots," with no public space immune from this violence. Further, the racial and ethnic makeup of those in these galleries generally remains unchanged—Black and Brown, male, young, and increasingly urban. This profile promises to expand numerically, leaving an indelible generational mark that will last a lifetime, which, unfortunately, will be short when compared to White, non-Latinos.

The method of death has changed but not the characteristics of the victims! People of color, primarily Black-Americans followed by Latinos, suffer a disproportionate onus of violence in our society (Zimmerman et al., 2024). Nguyen and Drane (2023) provide another perspective on how Black men are disproportionately killed by guns: "The impact of gun violence on this community is particularly devastating for young Black men. In 2022, one in every 67 Black men ages 18 to 24 in Philadelphia were killed or injured in gun homicides or shootings. In Rochester, New York, it was one in 50 young Black men. In Cincinnati, it was one in 44 young Black men."

The lethality of guns is only increasing in causing extensive damage to the human body, bringing untold physical damages and challenging the funeral industry for instance. The power of these weapons means that an intended target, and those surrounding them, will suffer pain and be "collateral damage." Their community, too, will suffer although media and statistical authorities will only focus on the direct victims, ignoring those around them.

The death care industry, in turn, is being called upon to make these bodies "presentable" for final rites and that is increasingly arduous, and in many cases impossible, particularly when young children are victims. Guns are the leading cause of pediatric deaths in the United States (Ordoobadi et al., 2023), so child burials are to be expected. Their families cannot view their bodies in the conventional sense for their final goodbyes as traditionally expected, causing even more anguish if that is ever possible for a parent! Children are so special that they have set aside cemetery sections for their burials, which, sadly, are expanding to occupy more land.

Urban Black-Americans have ascended to numerical prominence in the gun death scene, a status no group wishes to achieve. Canham (2021, p. 296) touches on an important historical aspect concerning mourning within the Black community with implications for the death sector: "Black bodies have been the site of devastation for centuries. We who inhabit and love these bodies live in a state of perpetual mourning. We mourn the disproportionate dying in our families, communities and the dying in the black diaspora." This legacy spans decades and centuries, illustrating the depth of this violence. The fact that Black-Americans are disproportionately gun victims has not translated into significant federal efforts to address this problem (Carswell, 2022).

The physical devastation of Black-American bodies, primarily of males as the intended targets, although with women and children as collateral victims, has continued with semi-automatic guns as a body crushing weapon, literally and figuratively. All gun violence brings emotions that strikes at the heart of residents of all ages, but particularly youth, instilling fear and sad memories for those who survive, with serious mental health implications (Francis, 2018; O'Neill et al., 2020). When these mental health conditions go untreated, it further compounds consequences for families and neighborhoods, now and well into the future.

Urban gangs and drive-bys bring a distinctive "urban feel" or "urban terror," and additional traumatic baggage associated with fear because they are unpredictable. This is done without regard for collateral damages, as witnessed with the deaths of very young children and older adults who happen to be at that wrong place and time.

Gun violence is a national problem that increases in significance year-in and year-out, with deaths by guns surpassing deaths by car accidents (Fears et al., 2021), a key indicator of the magnitude of this public health epidemic (Butts et al., 2015). The nation's health cannot be judged without examining gun violence, particularly in marginalized communities. Unlike the political minefield encountered in instituting car safety changes, eliminating guns and the violence they cause has proven elusive and an even greater challenge, more so in undervalued neighborhoods among youth and young adults of color. For example, of the 373 Philadelphian's fatally shot in 2023, almost half were under the age of 30 years old, with 17- to 18-year-olds or younger standing out as a sub-group (Adams & Marin, 2024).

A focus on Blacks, particularly males, illustrates how this group faces incredible challenges in staying safe as addressed in the following paragraphs. Pittman and Farrell (2022), for example, highlight how Black-Americans have this country's highest rates of gun violence: "The vast majority of gun deaths among Black Americans are gun homicides, and Black Americans make up the majority of gun homicide victims in the US. In fact, 83% of all gun deaths among Black Americans are gun homicides. Despite the fact that Black boys and men account for just 6% of the total population, they comprise more than half of all gun homicide victims." Clearly, gun violence disproportionately impacts this community.

Nguyen and Drane (2023), in turn, stress how concentrated gun violence is in cities particularly among their Black men: "Research suggests that roughly half of all gun homicides take place in just 127 cities, 13 driving the elevated rates of homicides in these geographies. In the nation's 20 largest counties, Black men ages 18 to 25 die from gun homicides at a rate nearly 19 times that of white residents."

Nguyen and Drane (2023) further ground gun deaths within a racial context, and in this case, the Black-American community: "Black communities—leading to tens of thousands of gun deaths and hundreds of thousands of gun injuries. The impact of gun violence on this community is particularly devastating for young Black men. In 2022, one in every 67 Black men ages 18 to 24 in Philadelphia were killed or injured in gun homicides or shootings.[1] In Rochester, New York, it was one in 50 young Black men.[2] In Cincinnati, it was one in 44 young Black men." The range of 1 every 44, 50, and 67 concretizes the prevalence of this violence. These victims had their lives cut short or if surviving, dramatically altering them physically and emotionally.

Black-Americans, predominantly males, are killed at nearly eight **times** the rate of their White, non-Latino, counterparts, bringing a generational plague to continue with a public health lens. Readers may argue that using a plague to portray this health problem is "over the top." However, it does a good job of capturing the wide devastation guns cause as a generational problem. A plague does not discriminate; neither does a bullet!

Forty-eight percent of the nation personally know someone who has been shot (Everytown Research and Policy, 2017), which compares to 45.4% of the country using prescription drugs. The former is a staggering statistic for countless households contending with this violence in its various forms. This statistic would be even higher for Black-Americans because they represent 15% of the nation's population but account for 68% of all homicide victims (Sharpe & Iwamoto, 2022). Post-traumatic stress disorder, most typically manifested through anxiety, flashbacks, numbing, and anxiety, is difficult enough to address without a corresponding pathologizing of surviving victims (Johnston, 2024), complicating access to services by those in great need.

These victims have social networks, belong to and patronize community institutions, such as houses of worship, which also experience the consequences of these deaths. These violent deaths are not natural occurrences! Their organizations get impacted in visible and invisible ways, but these ramifications, which often go unrecorded and unacknowledged, are profoundly felt locally. These "co-victims" will hardly ever be accused of having a sunny disposition; rather, their outlook on life will be more fatalistic, and equally sad, they may bring anger and a higher proclivity to engage in behavior counter to their wellbeing, such as carrying guns for self-protection (Ammons-Blanfort et al., 2023; Comer & Connolly, 2020, 2023).

The following brief description of an interaction between a funeral home owner and youth in a high gun violence neighborhood of St. Louis is gripping due to its sadness and youth sense of inevitability of dying young (Masters, 2015):

> We deal with a lot shooting victims. It feels like anywhere from one-third to 50 `percent of all the homicides in the city come through our doors... I'd rather see old ladies who have died from infirmities, because it has an effect upon me, burying these kids. Sometimes when you have a funeral or a wake, kids will wander into the casket display room. They'll say, 'Hey, man, this is what I want. Put me in this.' Or I'll be making arrangements for one of their friends or their relatives, and they'll say, 'When I go, put me in this. This is the casket I want.' It really, really upsets me. When a young person comes in and says, 'This is the casket I want,' he's telling me he has nothing to look forward to but a grave. I'm not numb to that ... People don't understand that I'm human.

Youth fantasies about the last moments of their lives do not capture the pain and sorrow that accompany their death for their families and other loved ones. The absence of hope, too, is a form of death and one that is contagious with long-term consequences. Death care personnel are not immune from witnessing the presence of this death storm with no sunlight in the forecast if youth are truly the future of their community.

The nation's economic costs, in turn, are staggering and arduous to grasp because of the far reaches of this violence and best viewed through a variety of prisms to appreciate their magnitude and range. Clearly, they are a major cost with funds that can be better used in addressing a host of other national problems (Gobbo, 2023). These costs are often borne by those least able to absorb them. How can we possibly put a dollar figure on misery? That is not my inclination to do so. Yet, financing must not be overlooked in any comprehensive understanding of a public health epidemic and the trade-offs that come with spending public funds. Thus, what are the priorities for limited funding? The following section offers a variety of economic views to help us to comprehend this viewpoint more comprehensively.

The Death Care Sector Defined

Few of us have not thought about how the death care sector is defined and the institutions and tasks that encompass this system of care and its place in society. Generally, we find out what we need when we need to know! It is appropriate to take a moment and provide a definition of the death care sector, although this will not be the last time that this definition will be addressed and further expanded in a nuanced manner throughout this book to highlight setting-specific circumstances. The death care sector can be conceptualized as a series of institutions and a system that addresses critical elements associated with death and exists in every community, regardless of demographics, introducing qualities of a universal system signifying its importance in society (Eterneva, in press):

> Death care is an industry that has been built on key principles of honor, ethics, and hygiene. For instance, when a loved one dies, there are several steps that are taken to ensure that their body is treated with the utmost respect and dignity. The clinical side of death care ensures that our loved ones are laid to rest ethically and hygienically. Being careful to ensure that our loved ones are handled humanely and hygienically is crucial to preventing the spread of disease and maintaining dignity even after death. Death care isn't just the technical side of death but also deals with the commemorative and memorial aspects of it. While these services typically go hand in hand, these two sides of death care are very different.

The death care industry is a part of the social fabric of daily life in urban communities but generally goes unnoticed until a death occurs necessitating using this system of care. In the case of this book, an untimely, violent, and deadly one at that! Last rites are arduous enough to begin with but the method causing death is a key factor in shaping responses. When death is unexpected and violent, it dramatically alters the significance of this action, arguably unlike any other form of death. This sector is also facing other challenges such as ecologically sound practices, high costs, and a call for greater personalization of services. However, in urban communities, gun violence stands out in the realm of challenges, too.

Parameters of Death Care Sector/Industry

The definition of the death care industry requires further follow-up for us to conceptualize this arena, helping in developing interventions. The subject of the death care industry is one that I do not remember encountering in my professional education or at professional conferences and workshops I attended over my career, yet it brings universal qualities, particularly for practitioners specializing in urban practice and research.

How many of us think about the death care sector as part of any community, let alone an urban one? I venture to guess that we only think about this topic when we have to unless you live in a high gun violence neighborhood where this topic has great saliency. It is not a topic associated with comfort and joy and easily overlooked in discussing major public health challenges. Yet, this sector unifies numerous social conditions causing premature deaths and are entrusted to bring "closure" for grieving families and other loved ones.

It is the final service ("*ritual action*") where we can provide for a victim, but just as importantly for family and close friends, and one most of us would prefer not to think about. If we must, it must be dignified, memorable in a positive way, and one we can be proud of and even keeping mementos of the event, which are discussed in this book (Hoy, 2021). Thus, it is an important and memorial event in the life of a family and neighborhood, too! A funeral reflects on a family's pride because they get judged by how they treat their own in these moments. It is the final sendoff, reflecting a family's lore and pride.

The term "death care industry" conjures a distressing image in most of our minds and it certainly did in my instance. I imagine that most readers probably have never heard of this term. It is a term that attempts to capture a broad sector devoted to meeting the needs associated with this final life stage. This sector covers a wide range of services, some obvious and others less so, because of the nature of actions conducted behind the scenes, but no less important. The services cover instrumental and expressive goals that aid survivors in coping with grief and exercising cultural customs.

Premature death and homicide bereavement, as per Baltimore's Black-American males, for instance, translates into increasing reliance on religious and spiritual coping in helping loved ones navigate the emotions associated with gun violence (Lee et al., 2020). Gun violence does not stop at a church's doors, funeral parlor, or cemetery. When it occurs, it signals a heightened level of violence that separates communities from each other beyond statistical accounting of fatalities and physical injuries, including trauma and the disruption in daily life.

Barrett (2023) views urban adolescent homicides as an emerging public health concern and a challenge for the death care sector. Jenkins (2024), in turn, identified four perspectives on viewing the family and friends of Black-American homicide victims from a multi-faceted standpoint: "(a) the experience with local law enforcement and the courts during the investigation of the homicide, (b) the immediate experience of grieving over traumatic loss, (c) the long-term experience of coping with traumatic loss, and (d) their current relationship with the community." I would add a fifth perspective—engagement and challenges facing the death care sector.

Engaging communities and their key institutions in addressing gun violence is certainly not a novel idea (Bieler et al., 2016). The key is having an encompassing view of these institutions so that no sector is overlooked. There is increasing recognition that eliminating gun violence cannot succeed without active and meaningful involvement, if not leadership, in communities crafting interventions. That argument is certainly not new but it takes on a particular urgency when death can be so instantaneous and violent.

Economics of Gun Violence

Understanding the economics of gun violence is essential in developing a better understanding of this phenomenon. We will, however, never be at a loss to find data on the economics of gun violence, as readers will see in this section. It costs the nation the staggering sum of $557 billion annually, or 2.6% of its GDP: $489.1 Billion in Quality of Life, $53.8 Billion Work-Loss, $11.0 Billion Police and Criminal Justice, $2.8 Billion in Medical Costs, and $0.5 Billion in Employment Costs (Everytown Research and Policy, 2017). This translates into $1698 per resident. Each death and injury costs $274,000 (includes criminal justice judication and imprisonment) and $25,100, respectively. For example, between 2000 and 2017, it cost Chicago hospitals over $447 million in gun violence-related services (Schaechter & Hirsh, 2021).

The financial costs of gun violence in the workplace have started to increase for hospitals, for example, which is estimated to account for 0.05% of their operating budgets and projected to go up in the future because of increased numbers of shootings in this setting (Everytown Research and Policy, 2017). These costs will be passed on to taxpayers for this and future generations. Although the economic consequences are prodigious, the non-monetary social and emotional costs are even greater and not as easily calculated, including the generational and inter-generational ("toxic cycle") trauma that it causes. Trauma severely compromises daily activities and life itself. Community histories and reputations also get shaped in dramatic and long-lasting ways.

Shootings extract a price beyond human suffering and the altering of neighborhood interactions and relationships. Estimates have social costs between $182,000 and $916,000 per participant ($p = 0.03$), or a benefit-cost ratio between 4:1 and 18:1 (Bhatt et al., 2024). These costs fail to capture how dreams are compromised or simply destroyed for the multitude of victims caught in a web of violence that can easily spread across generations. Gun violence is an intergenerational form of violence, with all of the serious consequences that brings for families and neighborhoods. The intergenerational consequence of enslavement comes to mind and a good way to concretize how the future of the Black-American community, in this instance, gets shaped, with vestiges of this violence ever present.

Cemeteries: Rest in Peace?

Cemeteries are final resting places for dead victims of gun violence and not scenes for further violence to transpire. Gun shootings in cemeteries, nevertheless, are generating serious discussions of having funeral staff arming themselves for self-protection, particularly in cases of burials with a high probability of gun violence occurring, similar to what is happening in houses of worship. This introduces a contentious option that generates further discussion and even debates in this industry (Goudie & Tressel, 2018):

> 'You know when we're being trained on considering concealed carry for funeral directors, and that's up to us for whatever reason—it speaks for itself,' said Eric Hoffman, funeral director in the Chicago area. Officials with Catholic Cemeteries have recently convened meetings to come up with new methods to deal with isolated violent funerals. Roman Szabelski, the Executive Director of Catholic Cemeteries, said they are talking with funeral directors, police clergy and others to come up with new strategies to prevent the violence and raucous behavior. He stressed, cemeteries and funerals are over all peaceful and safe places, 'This is a very small part of what goes on in cemeteries,' said Szabelski.

The above description involving serious deliberations transpired in Chicago, a city facing serious gun violence challenges as covered in subsequent chapters, including a case illustration in Chap. 5. Few readers ever imagined that funeral homes, cemeteries, and houses of worship would be active crime scenes, let alone places of mass shootings and casualties. Mass shootings elicit images of night clubs and concerts, generally places of celebrations. Places of profound sadness as gun violence scenes are new in this country and bears watching as they become more acceptable to mass shootings transpiring there.

Detroit (Cogan, 2021), in turn, has the distinction of experiencing a precipitous reduction in gun violence, with the end of 2023 reporting the fewest number of homicides since 1966, a reduction of 18% from the previous year, and a hopeful sign for the future of this city. This decrease is largely attributed to community investments, actively engaging members and institutions, focusing on residents with high likelihoods of becoming victims or perpetrating gun violence based on prior behavior. Readers may think that Detroit, as a result, will not have a shooting at a funeral reception on cemetery grounds. Unfortunately, that is not the case. In 2023, one person was critically injured at such a reception (Kelley, 2023). One, it can be argued, is one too many! Services, regardless, do not continue because of a low number of casualties. A "show" must never go on under those situations!

Funeral Costs

It may seem crass to discuss funeral costs. Not doing so would constitute a serious drawback to any comprehensive understanding of the challenges facing many urban families. These financial costs are a major burden on low resourced families who all of a sudden must pay out $10,000 or more. When funeral costs are discussed, we usually think of them as related to monetary funds. That is a tremendous cost to absorb, and families may have to resort to using life savings, borrowing funds, or even undertaking fundraising activities as covered in this book.

The Illinois Department of Human Services (2024), for example, has instituted a program to help economically qualifying families pay for these services for children killed by guns (Oceguera, 2024): "$1000 in financial assistance to support their basic needs as well as up to $1000 for temporary relocation-related costs. Eligible

Chicago families who lose a loved one to homicide can receive an additional $1500 in financial assistance to support funeral or burial cost." Destroying headstones causes added costs that are generally passed on to the family of the deceased, punishing them financially, as evident in the Boston case illustration later on in this book. Increasing funeral costs have shaped how families address final burials while balancing a range of demands and considerations (Woodard, 2024):

> We spoke with funeral homes like King's Funeral Home, Alexander Funeral Home, and A.E. Grier Sons and Funeral Cremation who say they've noticed an uptick in the number of teens coming in. 'A lot of young parents don't have adequate insurance or no insurance,' Grier said. 'It does put a burden on these families when we do come in contact.' Grier said over the years he has seen a 30 to 45% increase in the number of teens coming in. As the impact continues to weigh heavily on the community, Grier said they've also seen an increase in cremations due to financial restrictions. He said there is a big need to further educate families on life insurance and final expenses. 'It's not something that's thought about in our community especially,' Curry said. Curry said it's an issue she's working to change by opening a non-profit called Krosswinds in her brother's legacy.

Changing values spurred by economics is not surprising for anyone working in urban communities. These changes are no longer restricted to the Black-American community. I have seen this in the Latino community, too, although this shift is still in its infancy but destained to increase in significance.

Not surprisingly, there are other costs worthy of attention, as in the funeral business, for example (King, 2018): "While schools and churches generally have programs in place to offer support to their employees, no such services seem to be provided to funeral professionals. 'Sadly, no. There are no support groups other than us sitting around and talking,' says local funeral director and embalmer Robert Clinton. 'We're a closed society, but through helping families heal, we get to heal ourselves. We kind of become part of their family for a short little while and that's what keeps me going.'" This description helps capture the humanity of death care workers that most of us never think about and part of the challenge we face in narrowing the divide between these two worlds—the living and the dead. The costs of good violence deaths cannot ignore the finances in saying farewell.

Death Rituals

Rituals exist when they meet a need. Death rituals have existed worldwide since the beginning of time (Hoy, 2021). Viewing of a body during funeral visitations confirms a death, allowing attendees to connect with each other, which is also very important. When a body is destroyed by gunshots, making it impossible to view an open casket, a critical act among many cultures in the grieving process is undermined (Paul, 2018). A final viewing allows a group to collectively concentrate their attention on the victim, bringing a highly visual act to transpire in a culturally reaffirming manner.

Testoni et al. (2022) examine how Western (medicalized) traditional views of rational perspectives on understanding and addressing grief and loss have emphasized pathologizing grief responses. Viewing of a corpse is an opportunity point allowing mourners to connect with the dead in a therapeutic and culturally affirming manner. This process, however, has become more challenging by how a human body can be destroyed by high caliber weapons, making recognition of a body almost impossible.

There is a welcomed and open acknowledgement that death brings its own set of rituals deeply rooted in cultural traditions (Rumbold et al., 2021, p. 601): "The rituals around death are transition rituals. They move the deceased person from one space to another—both literally and metaphorically—and effect a change in the social identity of bereaved people that is intended to hold them while their sense of self changes to incorporate their loss." Rituals emerge and persist because they meet basic human needs, often bringing long-held cultural and family traditions. Interruptions of rituals, in turn, are emotionally unsettling, and depending upon circumstances, can cause great pain and anguish, bringing potentially severe individual and collective ramifications.

Families can encounter formidable barriers in viewing relatives killed by guns (Reny et al. 2020). As already noted, viewing a body is considered socio-culturally essential in facilitating the grieving process, but that is not universally practiced in the trauma bay. When a viewing is not possible because of the body's condition, it compounds the grieving process. How can it get any worse? The answer is yes! This happens when burial grounds are compromised and when we cannot look at the deceased, an essential quality of paying last respects. Seeking revenge for this violation, in turn, can lead to other injuries and killings of innocent bystanders, compounding a tragic situation to begin with for loved ones.

The therapeutic benefits of that initial viewing, and the ceremony that follows, are best appreciated in the moment (Garrido, Undated): "The ability to come together, acknowledge grief and loss, and reconnect with family and friends seems to offer healing in a way that more modern and mainstream contemporary funeral practices (such as memorial services held months after a person dies) do not." Thus, the importance of having a loved one "*casket sharp*" takes on greater significance in the Black-American community, although certainly not limited to this community and called by different names.

One challenge is ever present but may be unconscious to those confronted with the need to attend these ceremonies. Namely, the concept of thanatophobia, or death anxiety (Brady, 2015), which captures a state of mind whereby people experience an adverse reaction when they become cognizant of their own mortality. This is only heightened with providers of death care services, as with gun violence, who experience even more profound feelings. This fear can compromise serving those in need in an affirming and therapeutic manner at a vulnerable period in their life, but also keeping them physically safe. In the past, it was not a challenge; today, it is a challenge in urban communities with high gang and gun violence rates.

Black-American Funeral Home Demographics

Funeral homes can be considered to be at the center of the death care sector, particularly when viewed from a community level. As already noted, this sector consists of those who work with funerals and cemeteries, as well as houses of worship involved with religious families. Other dimensions, too, are integral parts of this sector, including elements that will be surprising to readers. Nevertheless, funeral homes and cemeteries play a central role and thus worthy of attention in this book. These establishments can occupy prominent positions as sanctuaries during particularly trying times within communities of color, signifying the essential role they can play.

It is important to pause and develop a comprehension of funeral home ownership, although this is difficult to accomplish because of a paucity of data on this important institution. Funeral homes, or sometimes referred to as mortuaries, funeral parlors or establishments, numbered 19,000 nationally in 2023, an increase of approximately 200 when compared to the previous year. This number is still lower than the 19,700 recorded in 2004 (Statista Research Department, 2024). Three large corporations own 15% of the funeral home industry, giving new meaning to the "funeral industrial complex" if this percentage continues to increase (Waters, 2019)!

The high numbers and percentages of Black-Americans killed by guns calls for signaling them out for attention in this section and throughout this book. The vast majority (89.2%) of Black funeral homes are owned by Black-American families or individuals, giving testament to them being community institutions. In 2021, there were approximately 1200 funeral homes owned by them in the United States. The average funeral home serves 113 families per year, or approximately 9.5 per month, and employs 3 full-time and 4 part-time staff. These are not "big" businesses by any account and can arguably be considered "small" businesses in the conventional sense of the term, but that does not diminish their significance for families in their times of need.

In Minneapolis, Minnesota, for example, a city that rarely makes national news because of gun violence, one additional neighborhood gun homicide each year caused 80 fewer jobs in the next year and illustrative of the broad and detrimental reach of this violence (ILJEC, 2023):

> These costs include camera systems, Plexiglas, bulletproof windows, motion sensor lights, bars on doors, security staff and other security strategies. There are also costs caused by behavioral changes by business owners and residents reacting to increased gun violence that reduce sales. These costs include businesses closing earlier in the day, residents avoiding shopping during night hours, residents relocating and people avoiding moving to the high gun violence neighborhoods. While the Urban Institute study looked specifically at areas considered 'high-crime,' increasing violence has been shown to affect low-crime areas as well, as fear of victimization harms business growth and development. (p. 3)

Patronizing local family establishments, in addition, help residents develop social connectedness with other residents, bringing often needed stability to a community. When residents restrict community interactions, feelings of isolation increase with restricted social investments in their surroundings. I mention this here because the funeral sector, too, is influenced by shootings.

Savanah, Georgia, for readers who are interested, has the distinction of having the oldest African-American owned funeral parlor. The Bynes-Royall Funeral Home dates back to 1878, although earlier in its history it did not serve the Black-American community due to segregationist practices. Black-American funeral parlors, not surprisingly, were considered one of the earliest and most successful small businesses in the Black-American community, bringing much needed stability in a turbulent socio-economic-political world in these communities.

Black-American owned and operated funeral homes are closing at a greater rate than they are opening, and this is occurring against a demographic tsunami within communities of color within the next several decades that show dramatic increases. Philadelphia, for example, experienced almost 30 Black-American funeral homes closing over a 20-year period. That city currently has 75 Black-American funeral homes serving 650,000 of their community, or 43.6% of that city's population. This decline is largely due to a lack of succession plans and a failure to reach out to other racial and ethnic groups. In gist, diversification of its consumer base. Gentrification, too, has in the case of D.C. and other cities, has been uplifted as key reasons for this decline (Black Enterprise, 2022).

Latino burial practices will differ from other residents such as Black-Americans, for example. Unfortunately, statistical information on Latino-owned funeral parlors was not possible to be located, leaving a glaring gap in knowledge against a backdrop of projected dramatic increases in the population. I remember attending funeral services of many of my relatives at Latino funeral parlors, so they have existed for a considerable period of time. Scholars have a field of study that will benefit from attention and creativity, awaiting contributions to the field.

Bereavement and Grief

We cannot adequately discuss the death care sector without attention to the vulnerable state of mind of those mourning their deceased loved ones. Any subject heading with the words "bereavement and grief" is bound to make a reader pause because it is a human emotion that we all can relate to regardless of our backgrounds and one associated with emotional pain. We need to pause and define bereavement and grief, two concepts often used interchangeably and find prominence throughout this book, particularly for what it means to experience gun violence at a final rites ceremony (Falzarano et al., 2022):

> Bereavement is, by definition, a social experience because it is the loss of a significant other. Grief is the emotional response to this social loss, manifesting itself with feelings of yearning and missing the deceased person. Thus, both bereavement and grief are inherently social phenomena that are strongly influenced by social, cultural, historical, and political forces. Cultural factors contribute to individuals' perceptions of and meanings associated with illness, suffering, dying, and death. The communal aspects of culture, including social

> norms, rituals, roles, and interpersonal relationships, influence the meaning attributed to and the experience of the mourning process—all of which vastly differ across cultures, religions, and racial/ethnic groups. (p. 696)

The presence of gun violence in causing a death, and the experiences afterward in laying victims to rest, is salient because of its psychological/social/cultural importance when the cycle of putting a loved one to rest is severely compromised. These terms hold profound emotional meaning and are bound to elicit memories that make us happy when ceremonies go right, and sad and angry, regardless of our situation in life, when they do not go according to expectations. These situations cause lifelong memories, but they typically do not cause further deaths and profound sorrow.

Grief, in turn, and trauma in specific, are two constructs often used interchangeably because of the pain they capture, thus it is understandable that many readers may substitute them. These two constructs tap two different circumstances or situations, however, bringing forth different outcomes. Trauma results in severe physical and emotional or mental harm if left untreated. Death, particularly when violent and unexpected, are consequences of such an event. Grief, or sometimes referred to as "profound sadness," captures this state of mind. It is considered normative because we all experience it during our lifetime, bringing a range of temporary reactions such as loss of sleep, lack of appetite, or failure to engage in festive activities. "Temporary" and "normal" comes to mind in discussing these two terms.

Grief is a human emotion that can unite us if we attend ceremonies that understand its potential to be therapeutic and can be counter-therapeutic if interrupted by violence (Clark-Jackson, 2024): "Since grief can be isolating, disorientating, and even polarizing, we often try to ignore or bury it. We don't want it taking up too much space or attracting too much attention. It can be a burden, and one that fills us with unnecessary feelings of shame." Although grief is a universal emotion, it has different manifestations depending on the socio-cultural group being discussed. Rosenblatt and Wallace (2021), for example, specifically discuss African-American grief and the importance of grounding this emotion within a socio-historical context that acknowledges their unique experiences historically and currently, which has largely been ignored historically and currently by social scientists:

> Why the neglect of African American grief? One way to think about it is that many who write about grief may assume that African American grief is not different from that of Euro-Americans. In fact, we believe that the assumption is even broader than that. It is that grief is a basic human process. So just as all humans breathe in the same way, all humans grieve in the same way. Thinking along those lines, a person would believe that if we learn about anybody's grief we learn about everybody's grief. (pox)

Although grief is a universal emotion, it is manifested differently according to contextual factors such as race, ethnicity, cultural values, and social economic factors. Urban areas of the country with high representations of different ethnic and racial grounds will witness a diversity of manifestations, challenging providers of services in developing culture-specific interventions. As addressed later in this chapter and throughout this book, grieving in public brings with it its share of rewards and liabilities. However, its benefits seem considerable (Clark-Jackson, 2024): "But there's evidence that supports that sharing the burden of grief in public invites others to aid in the healing process. It can also allow a stronger social resilience to discuss topics of grief and mourning. And it connects us to community in ways that may be able to enact change. In short, externalization and communal care of grief can be transformative."

Disenfranchised grief, as per Black-American boys experiencing peer homicides, which may be new form of grief to some readers, can cause increased anger or rage (Pabon & Basile, 2022), with guns providing a convenient but potentially deadly outlet for these intense feelings. This grief is typically not socially acknowledged and thereby unsupported by others. Their grieving can only be expected to be magnified during shootings at last rites ceremonies, such as at a church, funeral home, or during an actual burial, per this book. In many ways, when we are at our most emotionally compromised state of mind during these events.

Disenfranchised grief is what marginalized urban communities of color experience in our country. We can, of course, view this concept from an individualistic standpoint. The external world simply ignores the pain and suffering these communities suffer at the hands of gun violence, with the occasional news coverage that comes along when an act is considered grievous enough to capture headlines, and then forgotten until the next tragedy. In the meantime, suffering goes on without external recognition, eschewing by putting resources in place to aid them recognize this grief rather than just "getting over it" and moving on. Historically, unrecognized community grief often goes unrecognized and that can still be said today. A collective experience calls for a collective response.

Chapter 4 is specifically focused on community trauma, which is significantly different and takes a broader and collective standpoint on gun violence, expanding the parameters of this violence's consequential reach. This view helps us better conceptualize service delivery. Community trauma does not take away from the importance of other forms of trauma. It is a frame of view that does not prevent individualistic trauma from occurring, which is obviously very important. Scholarly acknowledgement of community trauma is relatively late to the trauma scene and much in need of advocates to further shape this construct's influence in this field.

Life Expectancy and Gun Deaths

Discussion of death elicits a range of responses depending upon the group engaging in this activity, the circumstances leading to death, and the religious lens they gravitate toward when present. Broadening the perspective to encompass a wider lens helps us appreciate dimensions not normally covered in the urban life literature, for example. "Urban life" brings excitement and adventures but also tensions and pain of various types that can severely compromise health and wellbeing. Life expectancy brings an important perspective on premature death, allowing us to measure its immediate and long-range impact on various groups and communities, with overlaps and distinctive views to better grasp the causes and solutions to extending life, and greatly influenced by context.

Readers must understand and appreciate that the concept of life expectancy we learned in school, and in many of our personal lives, simply does not exist in the conventional way in many urban centers. Life expectancy is significantly shorter in countless urban households of color throughout the nation. “Old age” may mean that one is in their 40 s rather than late 70 s or 80 s. Adulthood, with all of the responsibilities that it brings, may start in the mid-teens. Parentified children in dysfunctional homes come to mind capturing role reversals and the demands they put on youth, for example.

This “new” life expectancy viewpoint influences world views and how much time we have on this earth. When asking urban youth of color in high gun violence communities what comes to mind when I say “old-age,” I am always taken aback by the responses, and it takes a lot for this to happen to me. Asking this same question of youth in an upper-middle class community elicits answers we typically learn in our academic preparations. We must keep this in mind when discussions focus on life expectancy within and across communities, and when someone says that someone died “young,” That generally will be someone in their latency or early stage of life.

A statistical view of life expectancy, which is a popular way of discussing this concept in academic circles, invariably highlights genetics, lifestyle, diet, access to institutional supports, and ecological factors, with gun violence being one prominent influencer that has attracted increasingly more recent attention (Caplan, 2024). COVID-19, for example, played an instrumental role in lowering life expectancy in this country and throughout the world. In this instance, its impact was particularly hard in the case in urban communities of color.

High life expectancy is universally equated with a high standard of living, reflecting well on a nation’s goals, policies, and funding priorities, helping to ensure a healthy and long-life expectancy. It is a unit of analysis applicable to and across communities, allowing us to compare within an urban context. True, this unit of analysis is broad and often overlooks other key factors. However, it still helps guide policy makers in directing resources to correct significant imbalances.

Gun violence, nevertheless, wields considerable impact on life expectancies and a popular way our society uses to measure the influence of external factors on longevity and the health of the nation. For example, Black-American men (20–26 years of age) are 22.5 times more likely to die from gun violence than their White, non-Latino counterparts (González-Guarda, 2023). The probabilities of dying from gun violence is not equal across racial and ethnic groups.

A 2018 national study estimated the gun-related deaths between 2000 and 2016 caused the reduction of the average life expectancy by almost 2.5% (Samuels, 2018). Not surprisingly, upon a closer examination, one will see significant differences between who are dying “young” and “old.” White, non-Latinos witnessed a decrease by 2.23 years while Black-Americans lost 4.14 years, a 54% difference! The latter, unfortunately, were more likely to be shot and killed at age 20, and also most likely at the hands of another. It is imperative that when we view statistics, we do not forget to attach a human life to these numbers, including putting social networks to them because of how these lives lost impact so many other lives, too, and the institutions that they patronized.

When guns are involved, White, non-Latinos, not only die later but also by their own hands through suicide, which is not associated with urban people of color. Violence is responsible for taking a higher death toll on Black-Americans than cancer, stroke, and diabetes combined (Currie, 2020), introducing a different perspective on the frequency of violent deaths in this community. Death by suicide or health conditions deemed worthy of ending their lives will not be expected to have retribution on the agenda at their last rites, house of worship, funeral parlor, or a cemetery. Those at a non-gun related burial can be engulfed in a gun shooting and suffer consequences, further introducing tragedy to a solemn event.

Children and Adolescents: A Growth Industry for the Death Care Sector?

I am not fond of this section's title but it captures my intent in writing it. We usually think of an increasingly ageing population as a key group for the death care sector, and this nation is definitely aging and baby boomers are a key source of consumers for this industry. Of course, this projection is dependent on boomers having a life trajectory that conforms to what statisticians predict of an accepted lifecycle viewpoint (Delgado, 2014).

Nevertheless, it is truly a sad commentary to focus on the ramifications of gun violence on children and adolescents. This country has the distinction of having the highest rate of child and adolescents gun deaths when compared to peer countries (COVIDNEWS, 2024): "From 2012 to 2022, nearly 19,700 children ages 17 and younger died by firearm. During this period, firearm death rates gradually rose until 2017, then slowed through 2019, before sharply rising with the onset of the pandemic and holding steady in 2022 ... From 2019 to 2022, the firearm death rate among children and adolescents increased by 46% (from 2.4 to 3.5 per 100,000). This translates to seven children per day dying by firearm in 2022."

Estimates have gun violence killing the equivalent of a busload of children each week, vividly illustrating the toll it takes on children and their families and communities (Hoffman, 2024). One child dying is too much, suffice it to say! The same can be said to having their final rites services severely compromised. The death of these children has a long-lasting impact on their families and neighborhoods, as to be expected. Society, too, suffers this loss!

Making Sense of Violent Community Deaths

Social scientists often seek to answer the question of what motivates a person to commit a violent act. However, is it really possible to develop a sense of what makes someone commit a violent act of any kind, but particularly one that involves a weapon without regard for innocent bystanders, such as children?

Gun violence is generally reported on a national scale by major media outlets, shaping a national understanding of this public health problem (Henry et al., 2024, p. 68): "The local and national understanding of gun violence is often shaped by media reports that focus primarily on the immediate events surrounding gruesome shootings. Critical stories are missing from this discourse, stories of mothers who left the hospital empty-handed after the death of their children; of survivors of non-fatal gunshot injuries who have tremendous insights into what would have helped them to heal physically and mentally and to break retaliatory cycles of violence—if only." It is as local as it can get when we delve down deeply into who and where it occurred. Rarely is there similar attention to those physically injured but were "lucky" to survive (Delgado, 2022), nor is there any attention to the invisible wounds such as trauma.

Media, national and local, move on with the next day's news, but the ramifications of these shootings linger on far into the future and are a constant reminder of pain and suffering, and even for generations when discussing generational trauma, which is associated with enslavement but can also be applied to other spheres (Baack, 2017; Reilly, 2024). Local news coverage of gun violence shapes how the general public understands and views gun violence from a public safety perspective, impeding support for public health initiatives (Beard et al., 2024; Tourni et al., 2024).

Kolansky's (2024a, 2024b) Philadelphia study uplifts the importance of media not dehumanizing gun violence victims, including the tendency to overgeneralize across all communities, per the case of North, South, and West Philadelphia, because each of these communities has its own identity, challenges, and resources from the rest of the city. If the only tool we have is a hammer, then everything starts looking like a nail! Some neighborhoods may have more houses of worship, for example; others may have a high concentration of formal trauma resources. Neighborhoods are only equal from a 34,000-foot view.

Black-American suffering has evolved over the past two centuries with gun violence the latest evolution of emotional and physical pain (Harris, 2020), with what transpires during this stage of mourning. Successful solutions to gun violence will forever remain at the local level, but there is no question that it will require a national commitment, including resources worthy of a national epidemic! Urban communities of color do own or have gun manufacturing plants located there. Neither are they known for owning stock in these companies! The misery caused by guns is imposed from outside the community, along with other ills complicating the lives of residents.

The internalization of the code of the streets (Anderson, 2000) rewards outward displays of power through violence is a key factor in helping to shape the stance where there are no sanctuaries in a community (Burrell et al., 2021). "'The code' builds that might makes right and that if qualified, a person who needs anything may be moved to simply take it by force or stealth. Only the strongest, the willets, and most streetwise will survive, and so when people see an opportunity, they go for it." One key difference from 1995 and today is the availability of high-powered weapons. Using guns to manifest power and create fear is the latest evolution of this goal, with semi-automatic weapons ascending to even greater prominence because of the destruction they can cause in a quick moment in time.

A violent death signifies a death before its time and in a brutal manner with images that can last a life time for loved ones. It brings an end to a victim's potential contributions to their families, community, and society, including other anticipated and unanticipated ramifications. The gun violence field can respond in highly creative and participatory manners, such as storytelling (Gordon et al., 2024). Storytelling helps us address gun trauma by drawing on cultural traditions and the non-threatening nature of this method with the potential to reach wide-ranging audiences. Stories, when well told and using requisite symbolism, bring audiences to a destination they relate to, bringing hope, therapeutic outcomes, including potential action, too.

Other approaches, such as use of art (Efodzi et al., 2024; Nelms, 2024; Parham-Payne, 2014; Visser, 2021), music (Myers-Coffman, 2024; Stuart, 2020), and dance (Hyche, 2024), help communities heal, reflecting a range of creative interventions to mourning allowing local circumstances and socio-cultural factors to dictate how they unfold. Music, for example, is often integral to death care settings, helping us to center ourselves in a solemn moment and fostering an atmosphere of deep respect. Similar efforts are absent when discussing funeral parlors in high gun violence communities, opening the door for questioning and introduction of innovative approaches, which this book seeks to document and advance.

The gun violence field can never afford to stand still and needs to creatively expand to include community institutions that have generally escaped scholarly and practice attention. This is both exciting and challenging when it breaks new conceptual and practice ground. Breaking new ground is critical to urban communities of color because past conventional wisdom has not succeeded, without much debate on that point. That charge on proposing innovative approaches exciting and brings great trepidation at the same time.

Why is this the case? Death, of any kind, is bound to be a topic many of us generally like to eschew if at all possible. For some of us, it elicits memories of painful passings before their time, so to speak. For others, it may well be the mere thought of "losing" someone near and dear to us is too painful to contemplate. Regardless, the prospect of losing someone to violence will vary considerably between zip codes, introducing a completely different set of dynamics concerning death! One zip code has it as a painful reality; the other it is a mere passing thought.

Gun Violence, Death, and Threats to Systems of Care

There are multitude of ways of thinking about death with all possessing challenges when discussing gun violence, requiring countless professions and disciplines shaping their viewpoints in response. At its most basic level, death is a biological and life stage we face and the ultimate great equalizer in society regardless of demographic circumstances. In other words, we will all die, with the question being at what point and circumstances? Even in this final stage there are great disparities, particularly in the circumstances leading to final rites—the age, and other characteristics of the deceased. Although death is the great equalizer in the end, the circumstances leasing to it are not!

Gun violence health disparities bring yet another perspective on a disparity construct (Castater et al., 2024). These disparities invariably refer to a range of environmental factors that shape health behavioral outcomes, such as toxic exposures, for example. Ansell's (2020) book titled *The death gap: How inequality kills* lays out the consequences of this widening income gap using Chicago as an illustration of how poor health causes premature death and significant racial disparities.

Death can be disguised in various forms, some highly visible and violent, while others are invisible but can be just as painful for relatives. In the case of highly visible deaths, it is much easier to identify these victims and address their needs. Unfortunately, we cannot say the same for victims who remain invisible, which can be further compounded among those who do not speak English and are undocumented.

Guns have introduced a quick, highly visible, and deadly factor, particularly in urban centers and more specifically communities of color facing a host of other health and social equity challenges. Further, gun violence has disproportionately impacted youth and young adults, predominantly males, who are not supposed to die so early in their lives, introducing a dimension to a tragic event that no parent wants to confront. Afterall, parents are not supposed to bury their children! Children are the future of their families, communities, and society.

The gun violence field certainly plays an important role in helping us better understand the socio-demographic forces operative in gun fatalities in the nation's urban centers. These fatalities, as consistently noted throughout this book, disproportionately impact predominantly low resourced Black-American and Latino communities throughout the country, with certain cities and neighborhoods standing out by its devastation. However, in the process of painting a broad picture, we must allow for deviations to account for unique local circumstances because life is far from being fair and standardized, including urban communities, with each bringing unique or distinctive features, including histories.

The same cannot be said about the field regarding final rites, effectively ignoring a vital community segment and those providing services related to death. The funeral business, for example, stands out in this absence and why this book pays attention to them and their struggles to meet community needs while maintaining their health and well-being. There certainly are community institutions such as schools and churches, for example, with programs and services to support those seeking to help grieving loved ones, although there is much room for improvement and innovative initiatives in this realm. This does not mean that they have not established their own informal system of self-care and peer support. These efforts can be recognized and reinforced by the formal care sector.

Grieving the dead is a natural outcome over the history of humanity, with this act transcending private to public domains in recent times, as evident in public art and memorials (Visser, 2021). This movement is largely attributed to urban youth and young adults. Hoy's (2024) grief literature review (1985–2022) addressed three questions on Latinx and Black-American communities: (1) What are the grief interventions used with grieving two communities?; (2) What is the effectiveness of the interventions in reducing grief symptomology?; and (3) How has cultural adaption been implemented? This study found variations in approaches. However, there was a paucity of culturally adapted interventions. Further, the literature on Latinos was almost exclusively focused on medical complications while the studies on Black-Americans were largely centered on loss by homicide, raising implications for service delivery to these two groups.

A section in Cooper and Sciorra's (1996) book (*R.I.P. Memorial Wall Art*) made me pause and think of how a book almost 30 years old is still so relevant today. Although this book focused on New York City, it could be representative of numerous other cities across the nation. The author's note (p. 7): "Memory is triggered by contact with the objects and places associated with past events. This is one reason why so many who choose to remember set off on pilgrimages to battlefields, concentration camps, and Hiroshima's ground zero. We erect monuments at the epicenters of suffering and sorrow in order to appease the voices who demand that we witness to their pain and our horrors."

Artefacts tell an important narrative about the deceased, helping keep their memory alive for loved ones. In effect, they humanize what is often a statistic. Keeping the memory alive can also tragically cause further shootings and even additional deaths to those wearing these shirts, painting the memorials, or setting up and protecting memorial shrines. There is no end to this misery other than more misery.

COVID-19 taught us that grieving can take many different shapes, with online and drive-bys at funerals ascending in significance. Grieving, it bears mentioning, does not have to transpire in person as evidenced by the upsurge of online efforts used by Black-American adolescent boys, for example (Gross, 2023). Lighting candles at a church in memory of someone who is deceased is another example of doing so without having to be present at a gravesite.

Thoughts and prayers can transpire anywhere and anytime. These and other efforts have been motivated by a variety of reasons, one of which is staying safe but still having the benefit of a group to share these deep feelings; further, they are not bound by conventional holidays devoted to missing the dead in an organized and in-person manner. When grieving transpires in person and with others in attendance, it brings the power of the group to bear witness to this solemn moment, which invariably also brings cultural traditions.

The funeral sector does not have these systems of built-in support, with notable exceptions, even when they are increasingly finding themselves on the frontlines of what can be labeled a war with corresponding casualties. Historically, these spaces enjoyed reverence and the safety that goes with this designation, engendering a corresponding sense of respect and safety. This calls for bold new models to be introduced and modified accordingly to take into account a host of local factors. It would be a serious mistake to think one size fits all, although the commonality is generally a gun causing unimaginable pain and death.

These community businesses have generally been ignored in crafting services by the gun violence field, as if they were invisible to the consequences and playing a secondary importance in the life of a community. These places were considered final resting places and not battle scenes and "innocent" bystanders to this violence even when specifically targeted. This mind-set must change in any effort to confront gun violence in this nation's urban centers while expanding the terrain to develop interventions.

The trauma gun violence brings is generally applied to direct victims and their immediate loved ones, which is understandable. Those in the field need a wider lens to comprehensively capture these outcomes. A Wisconsin funeral director, for example, articulated the trauma facing funeral staff and why they can struggle with consequences to their mental state of being while attempting to meet the varied emotional needs of those attending their services (Peterson, 2018):

> Traumatic deaths impact those in funeral services, said Alan Creedy, former chairman of Wisconsin-based Funeral Service Foundation, which helps funeral workers build relationships with their community. He said those sudden and violent deaths cause additional stress for morticians. 'It's not just a body. Funeral homes are the ones picking up the body and seeing the aftermath. The body riddled with bullets and blood splattered everywhere,' Creedy said. 'They see all of it.'

This brief but vivid description uplifts the immensely important function that funeral parlors and their staff perform, with emotionally painful work experiences that cannot easily be left at the office, so to speak, when going home at the end of the day. The cumulative toll these experiences bring do not bode well for those who do not seek help.

Not surprisingly, there must be an expanding national call on who must be included in crafting supports and interventions because they effectively become co-victims even when not directly targeted. Bullets do not discriminate, bringing both physical and emotional consequences. Expanding this call to action, so to speak, brings its share of rewards and challenges as argued throughout this book. A national problem calls for a national mobilization and solution. Locally based solutions do not have national ramifications although they can certainly inform other communities across the nation over time.

Defining the death care industry requires casting a wide-net beyond funeral homes, also including cemeteries and cemetery workers, for example, because they, too, are often caught-up in shooting incidents as innocent bystanders. Cemeteries play prominent roles in communities, and we often overlook their contributions to society and how they can play a central role in helping us maintain a level of connection with loved ones who have passed but still remain a part of our lives. They have even been conceptualized as public parks and valuable sources of greenery in places where greenery is rare. "Peaceful" is a key word but unfortunately one that is less and less the case in certain urban neighborhoods that when combined, accounting for millions of people.

Clearly, cemeteries fulfill multiple functions beyond serving as final resting places. We can even think of cemeteries as green spaces in communities where these spaces are in limited supply, for example. In many ways, they serve as an oasis of greenery in a world of concrete. Nevertheless, cemeteries house our loved one's remains and home to important memories of our final goodbyes. Knowing that our loved ones are resting peacefully is a measure of reassurance in a chaotic life and are places to visit on anniversaries or major religious holidays.

The Mexican tradition of the "Day of the Dead," which can extend to one week, comes to mind when families and other loved ones gather at grave sites to remember and honor their loved ones through music, decorations, and food (Marchi, 2009), highlighting how cultural traditions shape how the dead are viewed and honored. When a peaceful state of mind is severely threatened by potential violence at a burial site, it brings a rush of emotions, all intense and negative, which can lead to further misery and despair, making cemetery visits and gatherings arduous.

Although this book focuses on gun violence as the prominent factor shaping the death care sector, violence can take other forms, causing psychological harm for the families of victims and those in this field. Yes, gun violence at these places is critically important for communities and society. Other forms of violence can transpire complicating the healing process and forever tainting the rituals associated with death, as seen in **Part II.**

Urban cemeteries are not restricted to high violence sections of a city, which may seem odd to readers with limited urban experiences. These cemeteries are increasingly found in the suburbs, as in Chicago, making them not immune from the spillover of gun violence (Goudie & Tressel, 2018):

> Police, funeral directors and cemetery owners are dealing with what they say are raucous and increasingly dangerous funeral processions that start in the city and end in the suburbs, a threat to mourners and anyone in the way. Most funerals and burials are reverent and safe, but sometimes the emotionally charged events result in violence. Police say the dangerous activity is usually sparked by gang retaliation... 'It's what we are dealing with now, I mean, they have taken funerals to a different level,' said Hillside Police Chief Joe Lukaszek. Lukaszek said suburban funerals for Chicago gang members regularly erupt in violence. 'People hanging out of the windows, hanging out of sun roofs, it just got a little bit crazy,' he said. The chief was personally involved in stopping and arresting four allegedly armed mourners leaving nearby Oak Ridge Cemetery. 'I saw a gun in the gentleman's hand that was driving the car. I just couldn't in good conscience let that car get on the highway,' Lukaszek said.

Breaching traditional social and cultural boundaries of where violence can transpire has reached cemeteries, signaling how the nation has changed regarding "safety or sacred zones." Safeguarding burial attendees introduces a new procedure that must be adhered to, but at what cost psychologically and financially for the industry? These supports cause increasing costs that will eventually be passed on to consumers, many of whom are challenged financially.

Why do cemetery shootings raise the question is nothing sacred in our society? Many of us have an impression of cemeteries as places that are solemn, sacred, and peaceful. That view is only a partial view of these spaces. It bears pointing out that throughout history criminal acts have been committed in cemeteries (Klaufus, 2021, p. 1058): "Cemeteries are desolate spaces at night and therefore prone to be visited by groups of people who do not wish to be observed to perpetuate acts of vandalism. Cemeteries are a common meeting place for illicit drug trading." Cemeteries have a long history of being places for unruly behavior. Thus, we must not romanticize cemeteries because such a view, particularly in the case of urban cemeteries, is not realistic, with the latest crime wave one example of why not. An attempted or successful murder at a cemetery is a new dimension on criminal activity, introducing the potential of law enforcement being present.

Readers may think that graveside shootings are the result of extracting revenge. Which, unfortunately, is increasingly the case. We must not, however, neglect gravesite suicides involving guns with scholarly attention on this aspect being traced to the early 1990s, for example (Danto et al., 1996). Graveyards have a history of witnessing gun violence, but there is no denying that the frequency in these shootings are occurring and their consequences, too, are increasing, and thus worthy of attention by the gun violence field. Unlike school shootings, the public does not have a worldview on this violence (Lee et al., 2022).

Cemeteries are part of gun battle scenes rather than final resting places for victims. In the case of gang burials, attendees, which often include other gang members in addition to family, are exposed as a prime target group, and easy targets when clustered together, requiring special efforts to be made to ensure safety for all attendees. That, by the very nature of the landscape, is arduous. Burials transpire in wide open spaces and attendees can be easily identified at a distance, particularly when wearing gang colors, with quick exists for drive-by shootings. We must remember that cemeteries can also be green spaces in cities consisting of concrete, taking their places alongside parks, for example, bringing these spaces more into the "life" of a community. This is paradoxical because these spaces are often viewed as "dead spaces."

There are countless others involved in picking up the body pieces, so to speak, associated with gun violence. Body Removal Attendants, for example, are invisible to the outside world and they, too, must contend with the consequences of personal safety and gun violence. In addition to contending with transporting bodies in horrific conditions, potentially leaving psychological scars in the process. Ironically, neither age group is associated with perpetrating gun violence.

Cann (2020) argues that African-American funeral homes, in turn, play a critical socio-cultural role within their communities beyond what we typically associate with this institution in White, non-Latino communities, signifying their enhanced importance as a healing institution and economic enterprise:

> Black Deaths Matter: Earning the Right to Live—Death and the African-American Funeral Home recounts the history of black funeral homes in the United States and their role in demanding justice for bodies of color and the black community. Through funeral pageantry and vigilant support for local communities, the African American funeral home has been central to ensuring that not only do Black Lives Matter, but black deaths count and are visible to the larger community.

Cann (2020) casts Black-American funeral homes into ascending to a lofty and significant influence within their community at a critical time of need for families of the deceased, historically and currently. These institutions are worthy of special attention for development of collaborative initiatives to strengthen relationships with helping professions and their organizations.

Funeral homes can serve as historical anchors in their community's history, with some in well-established communities with long histories of serving multiple generations and being part of a family's tradition. What happens when these "sacred" institutions occupying a special space within communities lose that legitimacy and are viewed as free game for shootings? Bunch-Lyons (2015, p. 58) addresses the unique position they hold within the Black-American community: "Funeral home operators occupy a unique place in African American communities. They comfort the living while burying the dead. As business owners, they are necessarily concerned with profit, yet their business demands compassion." They even have the potential ascend to community leadership positions.

The key word here is "compassion" due to its importance because it is so arduous to achieve when facing a life and death situation by simply carrying out their cultural, and spiritual responsibilities. Hazardous duty pay is not part of their compensation package! Black-American funeral home owners, by their very nature, have had to "be shrewd, and willing to make necessary sacrifices and to take risks." These personal qualities have not changed; the risks have changed dramatically, bringing forth potential deadly consequences in the process and causing a re-examination of continuing in this business and profession.

These institutions do not exist in isolation from the historical legacy of the Black Church, which often faces the same socio-economic struggles. The enhanced influence of these funeral homes can also be traced back to the post-enslavement period as the Black-American community was forced to bury their own, much in similar fashion to the birth of the Black Church meeting their spiritual needs due to segregation (Cann, 2020):

> Nowhere is the continued and persistent segregation in the contemporary United States still as evident as in the deathcare industry. First separated along racial lines during American slavery, both the funeral home and the undertaker mirrored the segregation found in houses of worship and the community at large.[5] Because enslaved people were initially prohibited from gathering in groups, [6] it was difficult for African Americans to host and hold a funeral for their loved ones when they died, and many early graves of those who died were unmarked or simply left untended.[7] Bodies of the enslaved were often buried without any kind of religious ritual or ceremony, but in some households, the enslaved were permitted to gather to bury and mourn their dead, just as they were occasionally allowed to worship congregationally. (p. 390)

These two institutions evolved closely over history and continue to co-exist, often in close cooperation and contending with similar external threats to their health and well-being. There is a natural alliance that can be enhanced in addressing the consequences of gun violence to their wellbeing and existence. Thus, an assault on one is an assault on the other. Unfortunately, both are under assault, making for a difficult situation and the challenge that much more prodigious for communities caught in this crossfire. When this occurs, its consequences are immense by the precarious situation they find themselves in meeting patron needs. Who helps them in their own time of need? Who is going to make the first move in bridging this divide, which can be quite dangerous in high gun violence communities? Do we have any other viable alternatives other than banning guns?

Readers wishing a comprehensive picture of the socio-cultural evolution of funeral homes should read Lampros's (2024) *Preserved: A Cultural History of the Funeral Home in America* (Johns Hopkins University Press). This book illustrates the evolution of funerals taking into account how socio-cultural forces shaped them in our history. I have never encountered anyone with an in-depth interest in this type of knowledge, although that will change as this sector increasingly finds itself in the news as a crime scene. It will then draw on the more intensive interests of academics and policy makers, but it must not stay there due to its national implications. Death care sector scholarship will emerge to create a body of work, along with a corresponding body of academics and practitioners.

This book only touches on this topic. Further, when covered, it focuses almost exclusively on Black-American funeral homes I was unable to obtain a comparable review for Latino funeral homes, signaling a new field of study that opens new perspectives on this growing community. Understanding their history is critical to providing a more detailed picture of its role in the Latino community, particularly when considering how cultural forces influence their role within different areas of the country, in similar ways to how houses of worship have been influenced. Cultural traditions, for example, can call for Latino families to wash, dress, and help prepare their loved one for viewing, which is an unconventional practice in this society. The saying "*If no one grieves, no one will remember*" comes to mind and why these objects when grounded within cultural traditions take on added importance (Prickett & Timmermans, 2022).

Further, families may elect to leave various personal objects in the casket, which historically it is not hard to fathom; most readers are familiar with ancient Egyptians burying loved ones with various types of personal objects. These items can be photographs or religious objects such as rosaries and pictures of the Virgin Mary, for example. What happens due to acculturation for newer Latino generations is unknown. These customs can be expected to evolve and change.

When a body's physical condition has been severely compromised, it will not be possible to carry out these Latino cultural last rite acts, undermining cultural traditions and complicating the grieving process even more than traditionally expected (Falzarano et al., 2022). When the only way a child can be identified is through DNA or the color of their sneakers, as in Uvalde's mass killings, it severely compromises this age-old process. When gun violence occurs at a gang burial or funeral home, this act undermines this entire grieving experience.

Gun violence has prominently found its way into these two institutions as communities seek to bury their loved ones and are at their most vulnerable emotionally. Thus, gun violence necessitates addressing it within the socio-cultural context where it transpires, with interventions taking into account the historical significance of these two institutions. This field of practice and research will broaden our understanding of communities of color and services, spiritual and social, for example, although certainly not limited to these two spheres.

Readers may think that funeral personnel must be accustomed to dealing with death and are therefore less subject to experiencing trauma, gun-related or otherwise. Afterall, didn't they elect to enter employment in this sector? The same has been said of trauma surgeons, for example, operating on gun victims. Becoming an active crime scene has never been part of a job description or a community organization's mission (King, 2018):

> A lot has been written about the impact of gun violence on our schools, children and society. But what about those on the 'front lines'? Funeral professionals and clergy stand witness to the most horrific experiences most parents can imagine. What effect does all of this have on them? 'When you handle services like this, it's quite heavy and traumatic for the families, obviously, but also for the practitioners,' says death resource educator and former funeral director John Christian Phifer. The job doesn't end when the funeral is over, according to Wesley Wright, a Nashville funeral director for over 20 years. 'Details of services for people over 65 seem to fade away, but kids who've been shot never go away,' Wright says. 'I remember everything--where they were found, how old they were, what their body looked like, their grave location, everything.'

Gun trauma is not a condition limited to mental health professionals and victim families. Providers of final rites, in the broadest sense, too, face challenges that often go unnoticed and unaddressed. They must be supported, as in the case of funeral staff, and often in ways unimaginable 10 years ago to maintain their safety and retention. If unsuccessful in keeping them safe, their establishments will close and residents must venture outside of their neighborhoods for these services.

There are many benefits for involving these organizations/businesses in community gun initiatives by broadening the parameters of what constitutes salient actors and institutions, particularly those dealing with a shooting's aftermath. Many challenges remain for those in the gun violence prevention field, including being shot or witnessing further gun violence, particularly those from marginalized groups of color, as experienced in one organization (Wilf et al., 2024, p. 34): "(1) being tokenized for their racial identities and experiences without having real decision making power; (2) feeling a burden to educate their white peers about the structural causes of gun violence and how to improve organizing spaces for other youth of color; and (3) being silenced in their racially conscious organizing efforts to address the structural causes of gun violence in their communities."

These challenges, when involving urban youth but not limited to them, cannot be ignored because they severely limit potential contributions to the field, particularly where staff of color find it challenging in carrying out their responsibilities because of their backgrounds. Another dimension needing further attention are the multiple traumatic consequences associated with addressing gun violence as integral to our work responsibilities, as per gun violence interventions. We do not have to be directly impacted to have adverse consequences.

Gun violence exposure among Chicago's community violence interventionists, although certainly not unique to them, raises serious alarms about the fallout of this type of work on their health and wellbeing (Hureau et al., 2022). These staff were predominantly male (84%) and Black-American (80.9%), with an average age of 43.6 years. Further, they were routinely exposed to work-related violence and direct victimization, with 59.4% witnessing someone being shot at, and almost a third (32.4%) witnessing a victim shooting. This work is dangerous in so many different ways.

There are various ways of thinking about the immense emotional toll (including forms of trauma) that gun violence causes during the final rites, arguing against a simplistic and mechanistic view of the dangers of attending these events. Trauma has been arguably the most popular way of characterizing this condition and its consequences. Corburn et al. (2022, p. 275) introduce the concept of "toxic stress," a condition resulting from a life of "frequent and sustained adverse life events, from an early age, without any buffering or support." When discussing gun violence, there is community support in various forms.

This graphic description of toxic stress helps us to visually better appreciate how your health and well-being can be severely compromised, making it difficult to cope in challenging situations and contexts. When these events were interrupted by guns, it sharpened our understanding of this condition and why it alters people's daily lives. Further, when they occur during childhood, it uplifts how a lifetime challenges awaits them. In some cases, post-traumatic stress disorder (PTSD) can be a consequence, which must not go unacknowledged and treated.

Experiencing a high likelihood of gun violence while on the job is not unique to Chicago, becoming an occupational hazard that many outside of this field may have difficulty comprehending and the toll it takes on them and their families. The closest professions to this experience have traditionally been the police and the military in active conflict, which should capture a reader's attention as to what is meant by "hazardous duty" in the gun violence field among this cadre of workers. Not everyone having grown up in a high gun violence situation can relate to this experience. Those in the death care sector are increasingly, personally experiencing high violence situations, with mental and corresponding health implications, and not to mention potential gun violence perpetrated on them for simply doing their job!

The goal of diffusing or interrupting situations resulting in homicides is embraced as a priority by the gun violence field. Understanding the spaces and events where retaliation is not only possible but also has the maximum impact when it occurs takes us where we can employ deterrence strategies (Braga, 2017; Wamser-Nanney, 2021), with the urban death care sector increasingly being one of them.

The increased chances of experiencing gun violence calls for highly specialized and multifaceted initiatives tailored specifically to violence interrupters (Corburn et al., 2021; Hureau et al., 2022), including rapid response teams and supports. They have a unique role in the gun violence field. Other high gun violence cities and communities, too, will find similar challenges for their front-line staff, needing expansion to include other provider groups, traditional and non-traditional. This necessitates new research and service delivery models that expand the terrain of who should be served and enlisted in shaping and delivering of services, reflecting the racial and economic composition of the communities they seek to serve.

Those in the death care sector have also be referred to as "last responders," quite a difference from "first responders." They unfortunately, undertake "dirty" but "essential" work associated with waste and death, and therefore stigmatizing (Kibbi et al., 2024). This makes it arduous to openly support them to begin with, let alone on a long-term and highly structured bases. Adding the consequences of exposure to violent deaths further makes them highly vulnerable to a range of mental health consequences. This does not mean that there are no current innovative efforts in this arena. Tan et al. (2024), for example, in a pioneering article on social work and funeral services based in China, offered a practice framework to engage this sector in service delivery, with applicability to other helping professions.

This is important for academics and practitioners because it acknowledges the unique needs these institutions address on a daily basis, introducing other service locale with them as key recipients. Further, our vision must transcend national boundaries in order to develop best practices. The United States is very different socially and culturally from China, with the prevalence of gun violence a key factor, and not to mention socio-cultural factors! Nevertheless, the field must not be bound by national boundaries because it expands the learning terrain for us.

This rather lengthy section on gun violence, death, and threats to systems of care has positioned readers to better appreciate how language can shape public perceptions of gun violence and who is to blame. Language, in bears noting, is embedded with significant symbolism, shaping our biases and marching orders, so to speak, providing a tool for meeting a host of challenges associated with this public health problem, as touched upon in the following section.

A Short Note on Language

This is a good time to pause and uplift for readers the language I use on gun violence regarding the death care sector. Words are powerful, make no mistake about it. How many times have we heard that spoken? The language or concepts we use on gun violence shapes public discourse on this public health problem (Betz et al., 2021). We can see how gun violence is discussed in the public media.

How we talk about gun violence and the death sector, too, gets shaped in a similar way. Words frame arguments when violence transpires in the death sector, introducing moralistic viewpoints tapping strong religious undertones— "sacrileges," "acts of violence towards God," and "evil," for example, standout. Unless used in a quote, I will not use these types of terms. I conceptualize these acts of violence from a social or public health perspective rather than a moralistic viewpoint. Mind you, there are moments and places when morality standpoints are in order. However, that is not my central stance in this book.

Book Goals/Methodology

This book seeks to straddle two audiences, practitioners in positions to implement recommendations offered in this book, helping the academy develop interventional models. The second audience consists of academics and graduate students in criminal justice, public health, social work, and community education, to list several professions. Academics and students are in positions to create much needed interventions relevant to urban audiences. This broad range of audiences makes it challenging to meet the unique needs each audience brings. Nevertheless, we all live in the same nation and struggle together, needing to breach professional divides to be successful, paralleling those in the death care sector and the formal health and social care sectors.

This book's five goals weave a variety of themes to produce a common vision and guidance for a new practice arena with all of the rewards and challenges it brings to the field: (1) ground readers in the latest statistical information on urban gun violence; (2) review existing approaches for preventing and intervening in urban community gun violence; (3) uplift the importance of the death care industry (funeral businesses as a major part of) in meeting the needs of families and friends of gun victims; attention will also be paid to how funeral homes have expanded their vision of services to aid their community; (4) a series of case illustrations provide readers with how to develop collaborative projects with systems of care; and (5) put forth community practice, education, and research recommendations for preparing future practitioners to work with the death sector to better serve urban communities.

The methodology used to bring this book's goals to life is multifaceted. I draw on empirical data from multiple governmental and foundation sources, secondary data analysis, theoretical synthesis of literature from various fields of practice and theoretical schools of thought, personal experiences, and information garnered from interviews. It is a synthesis that draws on my personal and professional life experiences. Every effort is made to uplift the voices of those most impacted by gun violence in the death care sector because their voices are rarely sought and heard.

Finally, this book focuses on gun violence as an act perpetrated on others, but it would be misleading that suicide by guns is a non-issue in communities of color. Black-American adults in high gun violence communities exposed to gun violence may be at significant risk of suicidal ideation during their lifetime, with an increased rate of suicide—witnessing an increase of 58% over a 10-year period (2011 and 2021). This is an alarming increase. In 2023, the Congressional Black Caucus (2023, p. 4) issued a report titled "Still ringing the alarm: An enduring call to Action for Black Youth Suicide Prevention." The findings speak volumes:

> The data are alarming—Black youth have the fastest rising suicide rate among their peers of other races and ethnicities. 1. Even more disconcerting, we may not have the full picture of how suicide deaths are impacting Black youth due to misclassification errors. In the 13-year period between 2007 and 2020, the suicide rate among Black youth ages 10–17 increased by 144%. 2. Black boys ages 0–19 have more than twice the suicide rate compared to Black girls of their age group. 3. In 2021, one in five Black high school students reported seriously considering attempting suicide in the past year. That same year, nearly 18% of Black high school students had made a suicide plan in the past year, and 15% reported attempting suicide. 4. Nearly 1 in 20 needed medical attention as a result of their suicide attempt.

Is the suicide rate among survivors of death rites gun violence elevated as a result? To what extent has witnessing family gun deaths and in the neighborhood influence this sense of hopelessness? Why not delve deeply into this dimension? These factors lack existing research, with the shadow of gun violence in their life possibly causing suicides.

Book Outline

This book consists of three sections and 11 chapters. **Part I**: Setting the Foundation has four chapters on definitions, history, conceptual parameters, and community trauma; **Part II:** Four chapters focus on case illustrations of various lengths on funeral parlors (Chicago), cemeteries and destroying gravestones (Boston), houses of worship shootings (Pittsburg), and a social media music video at a grave site (Jacksonville); **Part III** advances implications for the field (three chapters—research, education, and practice).

Case illustrations concretize key themes and are significantly different from case studies, such as a difference between an article and a book. Both can be scholarly but the level of detail varies accordingly. It is also the difference between a miniature portrait and a mural. Both are works of art but different. Both tell a story but the level of detail varies significantly, including audiences (Goodrick, 2020). Both have their place in the art world. The same can be said about case studies and illustrations. Illustrations enhance the value of theoretical material by applying concepts to real life situations. Various sources of information get weaved into a hopefully compelling narrative that facilitates insights, drawing implications for readers to apply in their own settings, and reflective moments. Further, comparing case studies can be arduous but when well accomplished can draw local and national implications.

Although this book addresses a wide range of U.S. cities, it has eschewed an in-depth examination of gun violence at funeral homes, cemeteries, and churches. These sites and institutions share commonalties on gun violence beyond being sites for last rites to occur. Nevertheless, each brings unique features worthy of attention by the field of urban gun violence in the crafting of interventions.

Each chapter highlights a particular city, following a similar outline, with documentation on gun violence in that city. The following section, in turn, offers details on a shooting or act of violence with an illustration along with commentary. Finally, a third section continues with analysis and concluding comments. Readers will develop a portrait to attach important consequences and theory. These final chapters offer recommendations for research, education, and practice.

Author Qualifications

Readers can rightly question the qualifications of a book's author. Ideally, an author must possess knowledge legitimacy on the book's subject, experiential and formal training. Urban gun violence has been the central focus of my scholarship over the past 5 years, in addition to undertaking consultation, presentations, and workshops on this subject. Gun violence is a complex phenomenon, and there is so much more we need to know, including yours truly!

This book is the latest in a series of books on urban gun violence I authored over the past 5 years, seeking to take a "pushing the envelope" stance: (1) Delgado (2019). *Urban Youth Trauma: Using community interventions to overcome gun violence*; (2) Delgado (2021). *Urban gun violence: Self-Help organizations as healing sites, catalysts for change, and collaborative partnerships*; (3) Delgado (2022). *The silent epidemic of gun injuries: Challenges and opportunities for treating and preventing gun injuries*; (4) Delgado (2023). *Urban Gun Violence: Empty Lots, Green Spaces, and Other Ecological-Focused Interventions*; and (5) Delgado (2024). *Urban Public Spaces, Events, and Gun Violence:*

These books broadened the parameters for urban gun violence initiatives; this book, in turn, introduces yet another perspective seeking to break new community practice grounds. Academics can advance new ways of undertaking projects. That is exciting, bringing immense challenges for urban communities across the nation and helping professions accordingly. Brokering these two worlds is essential if the academy is to be relevant in helping to solve this public health problem. To assume a position on the sideline is tantamount to malpractice.

Conclusion

This rather lengthy introductory chapter provided a destination, map, and marching orders, setting multi-faceted parameters on a subject that may be new for many readers but one that can elicit painful memories for those who have experienced gun violence firsthand. For those new to this subject, the journey will hopefully prove exciting and challenging, introducing new practice and scholarly vistas.

This subject is ever expanding, refusing to stand still to grasp its parameters and latest advances, much in common with an expanding universe. This is exciting and frightening at the same time, but there is no denying the deep sadness it also brings, including great apprehension because death is never a go-to subject to read about. For readers who have lost a loved one to gun violence, it will also elicit painful memories.

References

Abbasi, J. (2020). Large-capacity magazine bans linked with fewer mass shootings, deaths. *JAMA, 323*(2), 108–109.

Adams, D. & Marin, M. (2024, April 15). Philadelphia gun violence victims find support through residents and nonprofits. Wisconsin Public Radio. https://www.wpr.org/news/philadelphia-gun-violence-victims-find-support-through-residents-and-nonprofits.

Adeleye, A. J., Kristof, T. W., Naik, A. G., Laveaux, S. M., Cone, J., Faris, S., & Zakrison, T. L. (2022). Hidden trauma: Shedding light on the relationship between gun violence and infertility. *F&S Reports, 3*(2), 66–79.

Ammons-Blanfort, C., D'Alessio, S. J., & Stolzenberg, L. (2023). Self-help and black firearm crime. *Crime & Delinquency, 69*(1), 178–207.

Anderson, E. (2000). *Code of the street: Decency, violence, and the moral life of the inner city*. WW Norton & Company.

Ansell, D. A. (2020). *The death gap: How inequality kills*. University of Chicago Press.

Anstett, E., Duterme, C., & Robin Azevedo, V. (2023). Transforming funeral practices: Rituality and necropower in mass death situations. *Death Studies, 47*(6), 641–643.

Armstrong, M., & Carlson, J. (2019). Speaking of trauma: The race talk, the gun violence talk, and the racialization of gun trauma. *Palgrave Communications, 5*(1) https://www.nature.com/articles/s41599-019-0320-z

Baack, G. A. (2017). *The inheritors: Moving forward from generational trauma*. She Writes Press.

Barrett, R. K. (2023). Urban adolescent homicidal violence: An emerging public health concern. In D. J. Johns (Ed.), *African American males* (pp. 67–75). Routledge.

Beard, J. H., Midberry, J., Afif, I. N., Dauer, E., MacMillan, J., & Jacoby, S. F. (2023). "Like I'm a nobody:" firearm-injured peoples' perspectives on news media reporting about firearm violence. *SSM-Qualitative Research in Health, 3*, 100212.

Beard, J. H., Trombley, S., Walker, T., Roberts, L., Partain, L., MacMillan, J., & Midberry, J. (2024). Public health framing of firearm violence on local television news in Philadelphia, PA, USA: A quantitative content analysis. *BMC Public Health, 24*(1), 1221.

Betz, M. E., Harkavy-Friedman, J., Dreier, F. L., Pincus, R., & Ranney, M. L. (2021). Talking about "firearm injury" and "gun violence": Words matter. *American Journal of Public Health, 111*(12), 2105–2110.

Bhatt, M. P., Heller, S. B., Kapustin, M., Bertrand, M., & Blattman, C. (2024). Predicting and preventing gun violence: An experimental evaluation of READI Chicago. *The Quarterly Journal of Economics, 139*(1), 1–56.

Bieler, S., Kijakazi, K., La Vigne, N., Vinik, N., & Overton, S. (2016). *Engaging communities in reducing gun violence*. Urban Institute.

Black Enterprise. (2022, November 4). Here's why this Black-owned funeral home in DC closed after 80 years. https://www.blackenterprise.com/heres-why-this-black-owned-funeral-home-in-dc-closed-after-80-years/.

Boncy, A. (2024). *Changing narrative of gun violence*. Columbia College Today. Spring. https://www.college.columbia.edu/cct/issue/winterspring-2024/article/changing-narrative-gun-violence

Boschan, J. A., & Roman, C. G. (2024). Hot spots of gun violence in the era of focused deterrence: A space-time analysis of shootings in South Philadelphia. *Social Sciences, 13*(2), 119.

Brady, M. (2015). Death anxiety among emergency care workers. *Emergency Nurse, 23*(4).

Braga, A. A. (2017). Focused deterrence and the reduction of gang homicide. *The Handbook of Homicide*, 643–658.

Brigham. (2023). Semiautomatic rifles contribute to more gun deaths, injuries. https://magazine.brighamandwomens.org/departments/semiautomatic-rifles-contribute-to-more-gun-deaths-injuries.

Buggs, S. (2022). *Community-based violence interruption and public safety*. Arnold Ventures.

Buggs, S. A., Lund, J. J., & Kravitz-Wirtz, N. (2023). Voicing narratives of structural violence in interpersonal firearm violence research and prevention in the United States. *Frontiers in Public Health, 11*, 1143278.

Bunch-Lyons, B. (2015). 'Ours Is a Business of Loyalty': African American funeral home owners in southern cities. *The Southern Quarterly, 53*(1), 57–71.

Burrell, M., White, A. M., Frerichs, L., Funchess, M., Cerulli, C., DiGiovanni, L., & Lich, K. H. (2021). Depicting “the system”: How structural racism and disenfranchisement in the United States can cause dynamics in community violence among males in urban Black communities. *Social Science & Medicine, 272*, 113469.

Butts, J. A., Roman, C. G., Bostwick, L., & Porter, J. R. (2015). Cure violence: A public health model to reduce gun violence. *Annual Review of Public Health, 36*, 39–53.

Canham, H. (2021). Black death and mourning as pandemic. *Journal of Black Studies, 52*(3), 296–309.

Cann, C. K. (2020). Black deaths matter earning the right to live: Death and the African-American funeral home. *Religions, 11*(8), 390.

Caplan, R. M. (2024). *Long life strategy: A guide for living a longer, healthier, and more fulfilling life*. Springer Nature Switzerland.

Carswell, S. M. (2022). Have we surrendered to gun violence in urban America? Federal neglect stymies efforts to stop the slaughter among young Black men. *Race and justice, 12*(1), 126–140.

Carter, P. M., Zimmerman, M. A., & Cunningham, R. M. (2021). Addressing key gaps in existing longitudinal research and establishing a pathway forward for firearm violence prevention research. *Journal of Clinical Child & Adolescent Psychology, 50*(3), 367–384.

Castater, C., Jaeger, B. W., Hampton-Anderson, J., & Smith, R. N. (2024). Addressing health disparities in violence. *Current Trauma Reports*, 1–6.

Congressional Black Caucus. (2023). Still ringing the alarm: An enduring call to action for black youth suicide prevention. https://publichealth.jhu.edu/sites/default/files/2023-08/2023-august-still-ringing-alarm.pdf.

Cherry, T. (2023). *The trauma beat: A case for re-thinking the business of bad news*. ECW Press.

Clark-Jackson, Y. (2024, July 2). The revolutionary power of grieving in public solutions. Yes Magazine. https://www.yesmagazine.org/health-happiness/2024/07/02/public-healing-grief.

Cogan, M. (2021, May 1). Want to know how to reduce gun crime? Look at Detroit. Vox. https://www.vox.com/24145161/detroit-crime-statistics-gun-violence-rate-violence-reduction.

Comer, B. P., & Connolly, E. J. (2020). Correlates of school gun carrying among black, hispanic, and white male adolescents: Evidence from a nationally representative sample of youth. *Preventive Medicine, 141*, 106277.

Comer, B. P., & Connolly, E. J. (2023). Exposure to gun violence and handgun carrying from adolescence to adulthood. *Social Science & Medicine, 328*, 115984.

Cook, P. J., & Donohue, J. J. (2022). Regulating assault weapons and large-capacity magazines for ammunition. *JAMA, 328*(12), 1191–1192.

Corburn, J., Boggan, D., & Muttaqi, K. (2021). Urban safety, community healing & gun violence reduction: The advance peace model. *Urban Transformations, 3*(1), 5.

Corburn, J., Boggan, D., Muttaqi, K., Vaughn, S., Houston, J., Thibodeaux, J., & Muhammad, B. (2022). Advancing urban peace: Preventing gun violence and healing traumatized youth. *Youth Justice, 22*(3), 272–289.

Crandall, M., Bonne, S., Bronson, J., & Kessel, W. (Eds.). (2021). *Why we are losing the war on gun violence in the United States*. Springer.

Currie, E. (2020). *A peculiar indifference: The neglected toll of violence on Black America*. Metropolitan Books.

Danto, B. L., Taff, M. L., & Boglioli, L. R. (1996). Graveside deaths. *OMEGA-Journal of Death and Dying, 33*(4), 265–278.

Davies, E. (2024, January 20) He’s 14. He’s been to five funerals. Can he avoid his own? Washington post. https://www.washingtonpost.com/dc-md-va/interactive/2024/dc-teen-rashad-bates-gun-violence/.

Delgado, M. (2014). *Baby boomers of color: Implications for social work policy and practice*. Columbia University Press.

Delgado, M. (2019). *Urban youth trauma: Using community intervention to overcome gun violence*. Roman & Littlefield.

Delgado. (2021). *Urban gun violence: Self-help organizations as healing sites, catalysts for change, and collaborative partnerships*. Oxford University Press.

Delgado, M. (2022). *The silent epidemic of gun injuries: Challenges and opportunities for treating and preventing gun injuries*. Oxford University Press.

Delgado, M. (2023). *Urban gun violence: Empty lots, green spaces, and other Ecological Interventions*. Rowman & Littlefield: Lanham, Md.

Delgado, M. (2024). *Urban public spaces, events, and gun violence: Block parties, funerals, mother's day, and other community events*. Springer Publishers.

Dong, B., Houser, T., & Koper, C. S. (2024). Gun violence research from a micro-place perspective: A scoping review. *Aggression and Violent Behavior, 101951*.

Efodzi, M. E., Potash, J. S., & Moore, J. R. V. (2024). Supporting gun violence survivors with art therapy and legislative advocacy. *Art Therapy*, 1–6.

Egodage, T. (2024). Disadvantaged neighborhoods continue to bear the burden of gun violence. *Journal of Surgical Research, 293*, 396–402.

Eterneva. (in press). What is the death care industry? https://www.eterneva.com/resources/death-care-industry.

Everytown Research & Policy. (2017, June 23). Moms demand action. Everytown Statement of Purpose. New York.

Everytown Research & Policy. (2023, July 6). Executive summary. Inside the Gun Shop. https://everytownresearch.org/report/firearms-dealers-and-their-impact/#:~:text=In%20 2022%2C%20there%20were%20nearly,number%20of%20US%20post%20offices.

Fahimi, J., Larimer, E., Hamud-Ahmed, W., Anderson, E., Schnorr, C. D., Yen, I., & Alter, H. J. (2016). Long-term mortality of patients surviving firearm violence. *Injury Prevention, 22*(2), 129–134.

Falzarano, F., Winoker, H., Burke, R. V., Mendoza, J. A., Munoz, F., Tergas, A., ... & Prigerson, H. G. (2022). Grief and bereavement in the Latino/a community: A literature synthesis and directions for future research. *Health Equity, 6*(1), 696–707.

Fears, C. D., Dennis, B., & See Research Partnership Between University of Michigan and Community-Based Organizations Releases Plan for Improving Air Quality and Health in Detroit. (2021). A *report* from the clean air task force recites compelling facts showing that pollution kills more people than gun violence and car accidents. *Natural Resources & Environment, 36*(2), 45–47.

Fontanarosa, P. B., & Bibbins-Domingo, K. (2022). The unrelenting epidemic of firearm violence. *JAMA, 328*(12), 1201–1203.

Francis, M. (2018). A narrative inquiry into the experience of being a victim of gun violence. Journal of Trauma Nursingl. *JTN, 25*(6), 381–388.

Frisso, G. (2024). Children born of war: The recognition of children born of war in the Ongmen case. *International Criminal Law Review, 24*(1), 52–79.

Ganpo-Nkwenkwa, N. S., Wakeman, D. S., Pierson, L., Vella, M. A., & Wilson, N. A. (2023). Long-term functional, psychological, emotional, and social outcomes in pediatric victims of violence. *Journal of Pediatric Surgury, 58*(4), 774–781.

Gilligan, C. (2023, January 30). U.S. Remains an outlier in firearm possession, gun-related deaths. US News. https://www.usnews.com/news/best-countries/articles/2023-01-30/how-the-u-s-compares-to-the-world-on-guns.

Gillum, T. L., Hampton, C. J., & Coppedge, C. (2024). Using the socio-ecological model to understand increased risk of gun violence in the African American community. *Psychological Reports, 00332941241256635*.

Gobbo, A., 2023. The economic costs of gun violence in the United States. United States of America. https://policycommons.net/artifacts/4552595/the-economic-costs-of-gun-violence-in-the-united-states/5376158/ on 25 Apr 2024. CID: 20.500.12592/z4zv0k.

González-Guarda, R. M. (2023, June). Applying lessons from major public health accomplishments to firearm injuries in the US. In JAMA health forum 4, 6, pp. e232201). American Medical Association.

Goodrick, D. (2020). *Comparative case studies* (Vol. 9). SAGE Publications Limited.

Gordon, E., Gardner, R., Chéry, C., Sacks, C., & Masiakos, P. T. (2024). Collaborative critical making in higher education: A case study of a community-centred storytelling effort to transform harmful narratives of gun violence in Boston. *CoDesign*, 1–20.

Gore, J. P. (2024, May 24). Guns are killing young black people in rural America, too. *Word in Black.*. https://wordinblack.com/2024/05/guns-are-killing-young-black-people-in-rural-america-too/

Goudie, C. & Tressel, C. (2018, February 13). Suburban police, professionals struggle with growing funeral violence. ABC7Chicago. https://abc7chicago.com/funeral-gang-violence-procession/3073920/.

Gross, N. (2023). # LongLiveDaGuys: Online grief, solidarity, and emotional freedom for black teenage boys after the gun deaths of friends. *Journal of Contemporary Ethnography, 52*(2), 261–289.

Harris, J. H. (2020). *Black suffering: Silent pain, hidden hope*. Fortress Press.

Hawkins, R. L. (2024). Guns and the culture of violence in America. *Social Work Research, 48*(1), 3–7.

Henry, O. S., Batchu, S., Lachant, J., Armento, I., Hunter, K., Staffa, S. J., et al. (2024). Disadvantaged neighborhoods continue to bear the burden of gun violence. *Journal of Surgical Research, 293*, 396–402.

Hermann, P. (2023). Homicides are falling in many big cities. In DC, they're rising. The Washington Post.

Hitchens, B. (2022, July 26). *Second killings: The black women and girls left behind to grieve America's growing gun violence crisis*. Rockefeller Institute of Government. .

Hitchens, B. K. (2023). The cumulative effect of gun homicide-related loss on neighborhood perceptions among street-identified black women and girls: A mixed-methods study. *Social Science & Medicine, 320*, 115675.

Hoffman, B. D. (2024, June 1). Gun violence kills the equivalent of bus full of children each week. American Academy of Pediatric Medicine. https://publications.aap.org/aapnews/news/28854/Gun-violence-kills-equivalent-of-bus-full-of?autologincheck=redirected.

Hoy, W. G. (2021). *Do funerals matter?: The purposes and practices of death rituals in global perspective*. Routledge.

Hoy, W. G. (2024). *Creating meaning in funerals: How families and communities make sense of death.* Taylor & Francis.

Huesmann, L. R., Dubow, E. F., Boxer, B., & P., Bushman, B. J., S Smith, C., A Docherty, M., & J O'Brien, M. (2021). Longitudinal predictions of young adults' weapons use and criminal behavior from their childhood exposure to violence. *Aggressive Behavior, 47*(6), 621–634.

Hureau, D. M. (2022). Seeing guns to See urban violence: Racial inequality & neighborhood. Context. *Daedalus, 151*(1), 49–66.

Hureau, D. M., Wilson, T., Jackl, H. M., Arthur, J., Patterson, C., & Papachristos, A. V. (2022). Exposure to gun violence among the population of Chicago community violence interventionists. *Science Advances, 8*(51), eabq7027.

Hyche, D. (2024). *Grief like mine: A literature review exploring culturally informed grief work for black youth using dance/movement therapy*. Lesley University.

ILJEC. (2023. The economic toll of gun violence. https://www.jec.senate.gov/public/_cache/files/69fcc319-b3c9-46ff-b5a6-8666576075fe/the-economic-toll-of-gun-violence-final.pdf.

Imes, G. (2024, February 9). *Listening to Black violence prevention advocates helped me realize I was never alone*. Everytown Support Fund, 2024.

Jenkins, R. A. (2024). *The experience of grief, coping, and community in black families and friends of homicide victims*. (Dissertation,. Walden University.

Johnston, C. D. (2024). Grave preaching: Homiletical violence in the face of grief. *Theology Today, 81*(1), 27–34.

Karlamangia, S. (2024, May 29). This is how close we live to gun violence. The New York Times. https://www.nytimes.com/2024/05/29/us/pandemic-gun-violence.html.

Kelley, D. (2023, October 21). Man critically injured after funeral reception shooting on Detroit's east side. Click On Detroit. https://www.clickondetroit.com/news/local/2023/10/21/man-critically-injured-after-funeral-reception-shooting-on-detroits-east-side/.

Kibbi, R., Afifi, R. A., Pham, H., Sewell, D. K., Teahen, P. P., & Vander Weg, M. W. (2024). The "dirty work" of last responders: Occupational stigma risk and protective factors. *Journal of Occupational and Environmental Hygiene, 21*(3), 145–151.

King, A. (2018, October 1). The hidden cost of gun violence: Funeral directors | opinion. The Tennessean. https://www.tennessean.com/story/opinion/2018/10/01/how-gun-violence-effects-funeral-directors/1282437002/.

Klaufus, C. (2021). Safeguarding the house of the dead: Configurations of risk and protection in the urban cemetery. *International Journal of Urban and Regional Research, 45*(6), 1056–1063.

Kolansky, J. (2024a). *Gun violence in Philadelphia: Multidisciplinary analysis and A novel community-based intervention framework*. Thesis, Temple University.

Kolansky, J. (2024b). Gun violence in Philadelphia: Multidisciplinary analysis and A novel community-based intervention framework (Thesis, Temple University. Philadelphia, PA).

Lampros, D. G. (2024). *Preserved: A cultural history of the funeral home in America*. Johns Hopkins University Press.

Lee, J. R. S., Hunter, A. G., Priolli, F., & Thornton, V. J. (2020). "Pray that I live to see another day": Religious and spiritual coping with vulnerability to violent injury, violent death, and homicide bereavement among young Black men. *Journal of Applied Developmental Psychology, 70*, 101180.

Lee, H., Pickett, J. T., Burton, A. L., Cullen, F. T., Jonson, C. L., & Burton, V. S., Jr. (2022). Attributions as anchors: How the public explains school shootings and why it matters. *Justice Quarterly, 39*(3), 497–524.

Marchi, R. M. (2009). *Day of the Dead in the U.S.A.: The migration and transformation of a cultural phenomenon*. Rutgers University Press. New Brunswick, NJ.

Masters, K. (2015, September 15). "They say, 'When I go, put me in this casket.'" The Trace. https://www.thetrace.org/2015/09/st-louis-missouri-gun-violence-city-limits/

McMillan, J. A., Banerjee, S., Gonzales-Lagos, R., & Harris, W. (2024). Social factors related to gun violence in urban United States. *Journal of Medicine, Surgery, and Public. Health, 100155*.

Menezes, J. M., Batra, K., & Zhitny, V. P. (2023). A Nationwide analysis of gunshot wounds of the head and neck: Morbidity, mortality, and cost. *Journal of Craniofacial Surgery, 34*(6), 1655–1660.

Mueller, K. L., Lovelady, N. N., & Ranney, M. L. (2023). Firearm injuries and death: A United States epidemic with public health solutions. *PLOS Global Public Health, 3*(5), e0001913.

Murray, E., Williams, J., Lieberman, R. & Gebeloff, R. (2024, May 15). Mapping gun violence. The New York Times. https://www.nytimes.com/2024/05/15/briefing/gun-violence-united-states.html.

Myers-Coffman, K. (2024). Intersections of trauma and grief: Navigating multilayered terrain in music therapy to support youth through bereavement. *The Arts in Psychotherapy, 89*, 102166.

Nelms, R. D. (2024). Exploring grief and aggression through an adolescent art therapy bereavement program (Doctoral dissertation, The Florida State University, Tallahassee, FL.

Nguyen, A. & Drane, K. (2023, February 23). Gun violence in Black communities. Giffords Law Center. https://giffords.org/lawcenter/report/gun-violence-in-black-communities/.

Oceguera, R. (2024, June 5). How to apply for funeral and burial assistance in Illinois. The Trace. https://www.thetrace.org/2024/06/gun-violence-funeral-assistance-chicago/.

O'Neill, K. M., Vega, C., Saint-Hilaire, S., Jahad, L., Violano, P., Rosenthal, M. S., et al. (2020). Survivors of gun violence and the experience of recovery. *Journal of Trauma and Acute Care Surgery, 89*(1), 29–35.

Ordoobadi, A. J., Wickard, A., Heindel, P., Raykar, N., Masiakos, P. T., & Anderson, G. (2023). Quantifying pediatric gun violence by location, time of day, and day of week. *Journal of Pediatric Surgery, 59*(5), 1003–1008.

Orlas, C. P., Thomas, A., Herrera-Escobar, J. P., Price, M. A., Haider, A. H., & Bulger, E. M. (2021). Long-term outcomes of firearm injury survivors in the United States: The national trauma research action plan scoping review. *Annals of Surgery, 274*(6), 962–970.

Pabon, A. J. M., & Basile, V. (2022). It don't affect them like it affects us: Disenfranchised grief of Black boys in the wake of peer homicide. *The Urban Review*, 1–16.

Parham-Payne, W. (2014). The role of the media in the disparate response to gun violence in America. *Journal of Black Studies, 45*(8), 752–768.

Paul, R. J. (2018). Viewing the body and grief complications: The role of visual confirmation in grief reconciliation. In G. R. Cox, R. A. Bendiksen, et al. (Eds.), *Complicated grieving and bereavement* (pp. 255–274). Routledge.

Peterson, J. (2018, August 20). 'Not just a body': Wilmington's funeral directors grapple with city's gun violence. Delaware Online. (https://www.delawareonline.com/story/news/local/2018/08/20/wilmingtons-funeral-directors-grapple-citys-gun-violence/857626002/.

Pierce, O., Mascia, J., & Brownlee, C. (2024, March 27). You are more likely to be shot in Selma than in Chicago. The. *Trace*. https://www.thetrace.org/2024/03/gun-violence-statistics-urban-rural/

Pittman, S., & Farrell, A. D. (2022). Patterns of community violence exposure among urban adolescents and their associations with adjustment. *American Journal of Community Psychology, 70*(3–4), 265–277.

Prickett, P. J., & Timmermans, S. (2022). "If no one grieves, no one will remember": Cultural palimpsests and the creation of social ties through rituals. *The British Journal of Sociology, 73*(2), 244–258.

Puppala, P., Pick, C., Graves, J., & Harfouche, M. (2024). Youth violence does not discriminate: Inclusive violence prevention support services focused on counseling and peer support are essential for youth and young adults. The American Surgeon. In press.

Ralph, L. (2014). *Renegade dreams: Living through injury in gangland Chicago*. University of Chicago Press.

Ranney, M., Karb, R., Ehrlich, P., Bromwich, K., Cunningham, R., Beidas, R. S., & FACTS Consortium. (2019). What are the long-term consequences of youth exposure to firearm injury, and how do we prevent them? A scoping review. *Journal of Behavioral Medicine, 42*, 724–740.

Reilly, M. (2024). A critical incident approach to understanding credible messengers' experiences (Doctoral dissertation, Alliant International University, San Diego, CA).

Reny, D., Root, S., Chreiman, K., Browning, R., & Sims, C. (2020). A body of evidence: Barriers to family viewing after death by gun violence. *Journal of Surgical Research, 247*, 556–562.

Richters, J. E., & Martinez, P. E. (1993). Violent communities, family choices, and children's chances: An algorithm for improving the odds. *Development and Psychopathology, 5*(4), 609–627.

Rosenblatt, P. C., & Wallace, B. R. (2021). *African American grief*. Routledge.

Rumbold, B., Lowe, J., & Aoun, S. M. (2021). The evolving landscape: Funerals, cemeteries, memorialization, and bereavement support. *OMEGA-Journal of Death and Dying, 84*(2), 596–616.

Samuels, M. (2018, December 12). Gun-related deaths have decreased overall American life expectancy. The Brink. https://www.bu.edu/articles/2018/gun-related-deaths-decreased-american--life-expectancy/#:~:text=Their%20study%2C%20published%20in%20BMJ,nationally%20from%202000%20to%202016

Sanchez, C., Jaguan, D., Shaikh, S., McKenney, M., & Elkbuli, A. (2020). A systematic review of the causes and prevention strategies in reducing gun violence in the United States. *The American Journal of Emergency Medicine, 38*(10), 2169–2178.

Schaechter, J., & Hirsh, M. P. (2021). Caring for pediatric patients after gun violence. In L. K. Lee & E. W. Fleegler (Eds.), *Pediatric firearm injuries and fatalities: The clinician's guide to policies and approaches to firearm harm prevention* (pp. 143–155). Springer.

See, L. A. (2018). *Violence as seen through a prism of color*. Routledge.

Seitz, A. (2024, June 26). U.S. Surgeon General declares gun violence a public health emergency. AP. https://apnews.com/article/surgeon-general-gun-control-violence-deaths-murthy-24b53f1aaace068e0cb24ae809853f66.

Sharpe, T. L., & Iwamoto, D. K. (2022). Psychosocial aspects of coping that predict post-traumatic stress disorder for African American survivors of homicide victims. *Preventive Medicine, 107277.*

Shorr, K. (2017). *Shot: 101 survivors of gun violence in America*. Powerhouse Books.

Smith, M. R., Tillyer, R., & Tregle, B. (2024). Hot spots policing as part of a city-wide violent crime reduction strategy: Initial evidence from Dallas. *Journal of Criminal Justice, 90*, 102091.

Statista Research Department. (2024, March 21). Number of funeral homes in the U.S. 2004-2023. *Statista Research Department.*

Stuart, F. (2020). *Ballad of the bullet: Gangs, drill music, and the power of online infamy*. Princeton University Press.

Tan, W., Tsang, K. T., Su, J., & Zhao, K. (2024). Social work and funeral service: A proposed framework for practice. *International Social Work, 67*(3), 834–846.

Testoni, I., Zielo, A., Schiavo, C., & Iacona, E. (2022). The last glance: How aesthetic observation of corpses facilitates detachment in grief work. *Illness, Crisis & Loss, 30*(3), 336–352.

Tourni, I. C., Guo, L., Hu, H., Halim, E., Ishwar, P., Daryanto, T., ... & Wijaya, D. T. (2024). Detecting frames in news headlines and lead images in US gun violence coverage. *arXiv preprint arXiv:2406.17213.*

Visser, L. (2021). The dead and public obligation, grief, and action: A rhetorical analysis of the impact of invoking the dead in public art. *South Dekota State University.*. https://openprairie.sdstate.edu/cgi/viewcontent.cgi?article=1019&context=schultz-werth

Wamser-Nanney, R. (2021). Understanding gun violence: Factors associated with beliefs regarding guns, gun policies, and gun violence. *Psychology of Violence, 11*(4), 349–353.

Wamser-Nanney, R., Nanney, J. T., Conrad, E., & Constans, J. I. (2019). Childhood trauma exposure and gun violence risk factors among victims of gun violence. *Psychological trauma: Theory, research, practice, and policy, 11*(1), 99.

Waters, M. (2019, July 23). The death industry is getting away with murder. Washington Monthly. https://washingtonmonthly.com/2019/07/23/the-death-industrys-biggest-threat/.

Webster, J. (2024). Sociologic and psychiatric aspects of US gun violence: A cure for this endemic. *The American Journal of Medicine, 137*(8), 687–688.

Wilf, S., Reed, T., Millet, V., Ortiz, S. M., & Wray-Lake, L. (2024). "We been dying, and you got me on a call helping you stay alive": Black and Latinx youth organizers' experiences of racism in gun violence prevention organizations. *Journal of Research on Adolescence, 34*(1), 4–20.

Woodard, T. (2024, January 4). Funeral homes impacted by gun violence. WCNC. https://www.wcnc.com/article/news/local/funeral-homes-impacted-by-gun-violence/275-55e48953-1736-4a2b-a175-eb42324e03dd.

Yamane, D. (2023). Understanding and misunderstanding American gun culture and violence. *Journal of Lutheran Ethics, 23*(2).

Zimmerman, G. M., Fridel, E. E., & Trovato, D. (2024). Disproportionate burden of violence: Explaining racial and ethnic disparities in potential years of life lost among homicide victims, suicide decedents, and homicide-suicide perpetrators. *PLoS One, 19*(2), e0297346.

Chapter 2
Urban Community Gun Violence: A Multifaceted View

Introduction

I have a propensity to author books on "unusual" topics and enjoy stretching the boundaries of conventional thinking by venturing into topics few dare or are foolish enough to write about. There are few topics, however, for which I have to pause and take a deep breath before commencing to author or read about. Death is one of them! Death in urban centers takes that concern one step further because of the number of deaths I have witnessed and my affinity for cities—the bigger the better, as evident in this book! How goes cities influences, how goes the nation. This nation is urban-centered with its populations increasing by 6.4% between 2010 and 2020 (U.S. Census Bureau, 2022). We cannot exist without our cities. They must remain healthy for the nation to thrive because it is there where innovation and intellectual capital resides. Cities are not going away if we ignore their plight.

Death represents a physical state when viewed non-emotionally. I am hard pressed to think of a subject that can cause greater emotional reaction. Let's face it, defining it is not an academic exercise for many of us. Death means the same if it transpired in rural, suburban, or urban areas of the country! It is a universal outcome and fraught with a range of emotional content, cultural traditions, and beliefs, regardless of cause. Cities shape how deaths are manifested. Death is a topic that we can all relate to regardless of our own background and where in the world we live, often eliciting moments of profound sadness and one that manages to bring together people in pursuit of a common goal—mourning!

Death assumes many forms requiring the field to be open to how violence can be perpetrated on both the dead and the living. Destroying the memory of the deceased hurts the living and not the dead! The sections on destroying tombstones, taking and posting selfies or using social media directed at a dead gang members' grave (Chap. 7), for example, accomplish the same goals as destroying their gravestone, per the

© The Author(s), under exclusive license to Springer Nature Switzerland AG 2025
M. Delgado, *The Death Care Industry and Urban Gun Violence*, https://doi.org/10.1007/978-3-031-95682-9_2

case of Boston (Chap. 6). These acts do not involve gunshots but the consequences still take on an ominous outcome for those mourning their deceased loved ones.

Mass shootings have captured this nation's attention due to the randomness and causalities, causing increasing fears that these events are occurring more frequently and without any regard to space, place, and time (Fox, 2024). Visual images of these scenes make it easier for the public to understand the devastation of this act and how it can literally and figuratively tear families apart. Gun violence does not take "time-outs" or "days-off," and no hours in a day when gun violence is required to a take a holiday. That thought is silly to even contemplate. In fact, holidays have a greater chance of experiencing gun violence!

Viestad and Viestad (2023, p. 7) highlight how the dead do not leave us after they die and that statement has a great deal of truth to it: "There are two types of people: The living and the dead. The dead do not live with us. But we live with them. We dress them up. We erect buildings and monuments to them. We plant gardens in their names. In our towns and cities we dedicate parks and sometimes entire neighborhoods to them." Physical artefacts are subject to vandalism, introducing a new form of death to torment those left behind to mourn.

Deaths of loved ones can unite us in honoring and remembering them, helping us put aside differences for the occasions. Mourning can also elicit memories that validate joyful experiences; these memories can co-exist alongside painful emotions. Those who are very religious may embrace the hope of seeing their loved ones in an afterlife, reinforcing the importance of a religious ceremony transpiring according to cultural traditions. Providing the "proper" sendoff ascends to tremendous importance in these instances.

What caused a death and who witnessed it brings additional considerations and potential dire consequences for victims, their families, and those entrusted with their corpses, which can be extensive, recognizable, and unrecognizable. Regardless of standpoint and cause, it still is a painful and memorable event marking a significant moment in our lives. Some readers may go so far as to raise a death as a key developmental stage that brings a significant spiritual dimension that can easily be lost in a rush to find a practical "solution" to this final event; we must balance a variety of viewpoints to arrive at a satisfactory solution for the key players at this important event.

This chapter expands the terrain of gun victims to include countless others who are highly visible because of their relationship to the deceased and those who are invisible and behind the scenes in helping families and other loved ones to safely say their farewells. When the deceased was a shooting victim, death ceremonies transcend the usual boundaries and procedures associated with a "normal" death." Gun violence alters a depressing and even traumatic final rites ceremony by introducing the potential of further violence occurring at a sacred site and time, spreading feelings of sorrow and misery. Sadness and fear can often co-exist during these ceremonies creating a hyper charged situation.

It is not as if there is never gun violence at these ceremonies, and the same can be said for celebrations such as birthdays, Mother's Day, graduations, July 4th, and weddings, to list several (Delgado, 2024). These occasions, including the spaces where they occur, get negatively transformed and often in profound and long-lasting ways, reminders of a tragedy when a peaceful celebration was meant to transpire. In some instances, these transformations can cross generations.

Fehl and Mason (2024) discuss what happens when a public space used for a common good, as in the case of a marketplace, such as supermarkets, cafes, and restaurants, experiences a gun shooting causing injuries and deaths, altering the qualities that make these spaces attractive for engagement. These spaces are associated with daily activities, social gatherings, families, safety, and fun. Once they have a deadly shooting, particularly one with multiple victims, they get altered in a negative and dramatic fashion.

These spaces need attention and corresponding healing and restoration, too, for communal recovery to occur, which is critical to well-being. Delgado (2024) makes a similar argument uplifting the importance of public spaces for community daily life with the possibility of dedicating a permanent memorial to acknowledge a life(s) lost. Its application to the death sector is a frequent omission in discussions of urban gun violence.

An Overview Note on Funeral Traditions

A note on funeral traditions is in order to help ground how gun violence has altered this final rite. Readers will be exposed to a variety of funeral traditions in this chapter and throughout this book. It would be ethno-centric to equate funeral traditions as just another form of cultural values because of the significance of this final act Stanley (2016): "Black funeral traditions are distinctive from other burial rituals in American culture. Funeral directors have long preserved the African American tradition of home goings, as these Christian ceremonies are often called: Bodies are typically viewed in an open casket, and a richly adorned one at that, with large floral arrangements and ornate fabrics. There are limousines and nice cars to escort families, which lends a sense of pride and pageantry to the lengthy rituals." Last rites assume a form of pageantry just like other pageantries such as weddings, baptisms, and graduation ceremonies, for example. It provides loved ones with a public opportunity to show that the deceased will be sorely missed and is worthy of a "proper" sendoff.

When is a funeral not a funeral? Gadberry (2000) 25 years ago raised this provocative question seeking to capture dynamic changes in the field of death studies: "Change is an ever-present aspect of social life. Change can be swift and highly disruptive or slow and less unsettling. The changing structure of body disposition is an example of the latter. The traditional funeral is slowly losing the broad support it once enjoyed. This work explores three of the new methods of body disposition: (1) cremation; (2) secular, life-centered funerals; and (3) celebratory, 'fun' funerals." A fourth category, sadly, can be added to this list—funerals as gun crime scenes.

Secondary Victims (The Invisible Becomes Visible)

Although our society has a propensity to focus on the primary victim when discussing violent crimes, there are countless other victims known as "second-victims" or "invisible victims" who come into contact with the deceased because of their jobs and in the process become victims themselves (Gavin, 2023; Magee et al., 2023). They often assume low-profile or invisible roles to victim families and society in general, but instrumental ones, often behind the scenes but of no less significance in the journey of obtaining an external, respectful, and safe space (Reny et al., 2020, p. 556): "Deaths associated with gun violence are inherently different from those associated with medical illness. Not only is the deceased a cherished loved one, but they are also a homicide victim. 'As such, the body is often considered part of a crime scene... This duality of the victim's body—both deceased loved one and material evidence—can create challenges in terms of what grieving processes are allowed to occur in the emergency department or trauma bay."

A victim's body requires viewing from multiple perspectives, literally and figuratively, putting families in difficult positions during vulnerable periods in their lives and at odds with providers of death care services when their wishes are not followed. Death care staff, in turn, must balance safety concerns while carrying out their duties.

Doing well by a victim's body and their final wishes is critical from a loved one's perspective and not arduous to envision; it can, nevertheless, also put them at odds with the perpetrators of the death in the case of gun violence. This precarious position introduces a new dimension to gun violence where there are no "off-limits" on who can be shot and the circumstances when and where this can transpire.

Traditional boundaries simply cease to exist ushering in a "Wild West" mentality. Loved ones are forced to consider further harm versus "doing right" by the deceased, including going against their last wishes and not allowing them to publicly demonstrate their sentiments for fear of retaliation. This puts them at odds with attendees, further causing pain at a solemn moment and possibly causing future strained relationships. There are circumstances where mourners enter sacred places armed in case of violence occurring. Yes, they can bring flowers while arming themselves!

Providers of final services are often invisible to the outside world and the challenges that they face in carrying out their responsibilities. Their invisibility becomes visible only when something goes dramatically wrong, and when they, too, become victims of violence. The recognition of their unique position is a critical first step in the long journey toward service delivery to this cadre of providers. That is a tragedy within a tragedy, so to speak, yet one we are all too familiar with in many of this nation's urban communities, but generally invisible to outsiders of these neighborhoods.

The helping profession fields are challenged with how best to do their job in reaching this new sector once they realize its significance. Those in the academy, too, face hurdles of writing and undertaking research on this subject. Balancing the needs of attendees and providers is a difficult undertaking, particularly when the academy ventures into uncharted waters, which can also bring danger. These are not situations we strive to find ourselves in for moving forward with bold new ideas. In many ways, these contentious situations conjure images of wartime correspondents or researchers with similar stressors and potentially dangerous situations (Neville et al., 2020). This is done by those in the death care sector without the acknowledgement and prestige that these individuals possess.

The longer this challenge goes unrecognized by formal care providers, including the academy, the more dramatic the short- and long-term consequences will be. In turn, there is a greater need for highly concentrated attention and resources to their unique plights, with corresponding resources commensurate with the problem. These worlds can no longer co-exist in isolation from each other because the consequences of not coordinating them are just too great. For readers who are religious, there is a "third world," too, one that is metaphysical!

Rather, they must coordinate efforts to be effective in meeting the varied and complex needs of high gun violence communities and their victims. A failure to bridge these two worlds, creating safe passage to the afterlife for the dead and for those attending to get back home safely after a ceremony, only causes more pain to what is a horrendous situation to begin with. It also presents greater challenges down the road typified with what can be expected when we ignore a significant problem. Denial is not an option because it will not go away on its own. In fact, it will only get worse, similar to any infection, and it is a deadly one at that!

Shift in Paradigm on Who Needs Specific Attention and Services

We need to shift paradigms as we visit the topic of the death care sector. A discussion of paradigms, however, may elicit a load yawn or a feeling of dread from some readers, but is critical to do so. A paradigm is best summarized as a way of thinking, viewing, or a set of ideas, including values, clustering together to shape a world view. This is extremely important because it sets our marching orders, so to speak. A deficit perspective brings a propensity to only identify what is missing or wrong; an assets perspective, in turn, identifies strengths and resources in a sea of needs and misery. Community assessments must endeavor to identify assets because no community with an absence of indigenous resources exist (Parsons et al., 2023). This recommendation, out of all the recommendations put forth throughout this book, is the least likely to attract needed funding because of external biases that high violence communities do not possess inherent strengths or assets.

Shifting paradigms is never for the faint of heart and I say that most sincerely! Why? So much of what we know about the consequences of gun fatalities is grounded in the "formal" care services arenas; that is understandable because of the resources and attention our society has put into this sector. For example, burnout, also known as "compassion fatigue," not surprisingly, is familiar to helping professions. We can also argue that informal helpers as found in low resourced communities, too, face a similar challenge without much needed support.

Although hospitals are known for giving and sustaining life, often enjoying well-deserved public support in cases where they have been highly responsive, there is an obvious close relationship between hospitals and deaths. Patient deaths bring consequences that supervisory staff must be attuned to prevent emotional harm and turnover of staff (Boerner et al., 2017), as discussed in the next section. This consequentially undermines service delivery, compromising the mission of hospitals and the communities they serve.

"We Have A Right to Arm Ourselves!" Gun ownership brings intense national debates, including controversial Supreme Court decisions favoring the gun industry. "The right to bear arms" is a slogan that strikes at the heart of what some Americans consider their constitutional right with roots in this country's Revolutionary War. This "right" entered into new arenas that 15–20 years ago, we would not have thought impossible. Foreman (2024) further grounds guns within the history of this country: "Guns fulfilled an essential role in American frontier life, used for protection and as tools to dominate and conquer a continent. America's Wild West period became the stuff of legends as have the minutemen, sheriffs, cops, and organized crime figures. Gangsters and lawmen are lionized by popular culture and violence is commonplace in our media. Our society has fostered an American persona where guns play a mythologized role."

Houses of worship standout in this new frontier. Increasing numbers of church shootings across the nation over the past decade has raised alarm. It has raised security concerns due to the possibility of a stray bullet hitting a passerby and not an intended target. Just as importantly, it also raised contentious questions about conventional boundaries and what are "legitimate" places to attempt and succeed in killing people.

Although there is no disputing the value of enhancing church security, it is being experienced in other death care sectors. However, arming or not arming members has been raised along with other expected disputes on this strategy, and the message it sends to members seeking peaceful and spiritual spaces in their lives. Some houses of worship utilize armed congregants as a security measure, illustrating gun violence's reach and how it crosses boundaries normally considered sacred, safe spiritually and physically (Earls, 2023): "Numerous fatal shootings have occurred at churches in recent years. In March, an armed assailant killed six people at The Covenant School, a Christian school in Nashville, Tenn. Shootings have also occurred at other places of worship like Jewish synagogues and Sikh temples. When asked about their protocols when they gather for worship, around 4 in 5 US Protestant pastors (81%) say their church has some type of security measure in place, according to a study from Lifeway Research."

Using congregational members as a protection squad, and an integral part of services, increases the likelihood of congregants being accidently injured or killed when these armed members do not have the requisite training to use firearms in a crowded setting, in addition to engendering fears of violence occurring during services. A critic can label these groups as "church gangs with God's blessings." I have even heard them called "God's Squad." There is something fundamentally wrong for a society when arming God's House is considered a promising strategy.

These institutions are supposed to be safe spiritually and physically. One is not possible without the other. Most importantly, this stance on houses of worship security further escalates fears of potential deadly violence, which is ever constant and can result in an emotionally draining experience. It also engenders feelings of hopelessness and despair. In some urban communities navigating going to church is fraught with challenges to health and wellbeing when these institutions are located in disputed territories of various kinds.

Now, getting to church is no guarantee of safety once there, spiritually or physically! That situation is no longer unthinkable. The one exalted institution that was considered safe and where we could seek solace at any time is no more, leaving part of certain high violence communities without any sanctuaries to seek refuge. This is a serious gap in religious households that cannot be minimized, particularly as this deadly situation radiates throughout a community intruding into critical public spaces and public institutions.

Weapon detection systems in houses of worship, too, have actively been discussed in religious circles and another key indicator of how far the subject of gun violence in houses of worship has come (Gips, 2023). Where will it be a decade from now? A recent survey of pastors found them most likely to note that their house of worship has a plan for an active shooter situation with 57% stating so and 54% noting that armed church members are integral to the measures they have instituted (Earls, 2023).

Weapon detector systems are associated with high-risk settings and not places associated with God and good will. If God's home is not safe, where is it safe? When we combine weapon detectors with armed guards, it conjures images more in common with a prison or airport security than a House of the Lord. Active shooter training, too, brings added and intensely emotional reactions from congregants (Watts, Jr., 2024). Mind you, these systems were not originally developed to protect houses of worship.

These structures, with many entrances, pose significant challenges for these systems. The case illustration of a church shooting in Pittsburg, PA (Chap. 7), had shooters waiting outside of the church and then entering, sitting down, and patiently waiting before the shooting transpired within and carried outside of the church. Security systems, in turn, necessitate substantial money outlays and for upkeeping, drawing from increasingly dwindling financial resources that can find better uses for other worthwhile community purposes. I contend that these systems provide a sense of security, which may be a false sense at that!

Other society institutions, too, are rethinking their vulnerabilities to gun violence, such as hospitals and schools, with the latter getting attention because of mass shootings and murders. These shootings have attracted high media coverage because they involve children and high numbers of casualties, such as Uvalde's Robb Elementary School. Uvalde will be addressed again because of its significance for the death care sector, particularly because young children were the primary victims (Kellner, 2022). When the Uvalde shootings occurred, there were other mass shootings that did get national attention due to the magnitude and nature of so many children being killed (Montini, 2022).

Hospitals, too, historically occupied a highly privileged position in society as healing sites and sanctuaries from violence of any kind, but particularly its emergency rooms and gun trauma centers (Ryan, 2022). That is no longer the case, raising a desperate call for strategies specifically tailored to keeping these places safe, too (Adashi & Cohen, 2022; STAT. News, 2023). Hospitals share many similarities with churches and the death care sector because they, too, were not designed to guard against gun violence and were considered to be "safe." Now they can find themselves instituting gun violence protocols, bringing inherent vulnerabilities because of their physical structure (Evans, 2023).

Urban communal spaces often have the primary goal to be welcoming, respectful, and safe, taking on added significance because of a general absence of green and other spaces (Delgado, 2024). These spaces fulfill multiple goals for making life more communal, allowing for social interactions that connect residents with each other in a manner conducive to wellbeing. We can appreciate the important role these spaces play or have played in our lives, particularly for those of us who grew up in urban environments.

Communal spaces, in turn, lend themselves to hosting crowds and celebrations, making violence in these spaces that much consequential. When a sacred space is violated, it necessitates a special response commensurate with the importance of the space and occasion that is tarnished (Riley, 2024). "Business as usual" is doomed to fail and may even make the situation worse—adding insult to injury, by reinforcing a sense that no one in authority really cares what happens to them as long as they continue to kill each other. Justice is dependent upon them to exercise it and a recipe for further violence.

When undertaking innovative approaches, particularly when the subject is highly emotional and distressing, it is important to acknowledge that we are venturing into unchartered territory, with all the trepidation and excitement that such a venture brings. Yet, there is no denying that we must push the envelope for the sake of community wellbeing, and we can no longer standby and wish for the best without doing something to ensure that the best is achievable. Wishing it so does not make it so.

This book's final three chapters offer research, education, and practice recommendations for the field. These recommendations will not come as any great surprise to readers as addressed throughout earlier portions of this book. My hope is that readers become energized to carry out many of these recommendations at the local level.

The academy, I am afraid of saying, is often generally too reluctant to undertake bold ways of thinking of phenomenon such as urban gun violence and the death care industry, even though I have always considered that to be part of my mission. Maintaining a status quo is not what the academy should be about. Some readers may argue that this is not true. I welcome the challenge and hope to lose this debate! The academy needs the community and the community needs the academy. They do not exist in parallel universes. At times they seem to be so to the detriment of urban communities.

Communities know their own needs and circumstances, including who must be at the decision-making table. Professionals bring knowledge, so I do not want to minimize this. The saying "nothing about us without us" comes to mind on who should be at the table in solving any community problem or dilemma. This partnership increases the odds that the end result addresses community and institutional needs. Maximizing available resources is critical in achieving positive change, particularly in low resourced communities. How we conceptualize these resources is critical. Resources can be formal and informal.

We generally have a view of public safety with universal qualities, but these views are greatly dependent on the context in which it is viewed. Public safety matters in resource-challenged communities as well as in resource-rich communities. There is no disputing the devastating toll compromised public safety takes on low resourced communities, influencing resident worldviews, lifestyles, and outlooks on life itself. Attitudes such as the outside world does not care, or it is up to us to protect ourselves and administer justice, makes external interventions more difficult to undertake. Important scholarship exists on Black-American attitudes toward death and dying, for example, and funeral rites traced back to the early 1990s (Barrett, 2020a,b). Nevertheless, much work remains as the expansion of gun violence has taken greater hold since then, which can also be said for Latinos. We need to re-shift our views and expectations of the death care sector, as argued in this section.

Funeral Businesses: A Multifaceted Perspective

Few readers, I imagine, have devoted considered time and energy to studying the funeral business. Businesses are in the "business" of making profits. That is their bottom-line! Failure to achieve this goal means that they suffer a different form of death. The death care sector is different from any other business, although, they, too, must contend with economic forces to be successful or be forced to die, too. However, the death care industry recognizes that it is important to make a profit but also reach out and get further connected with their respective communities because of their proximity to violence and its consequences. They not only live with the problem but will also live with the solutions. If these solutions are unsuccessful, they will continue to live with the deadly consequences. That is the sad reality. Deaths are good for business. The nature of the death, however, brings its own set of challenges for this sector.

I would venture to say, based on impressions over the past two decades but not empirical evidence, mind you, that these small businesses have historically been family businesses, passed from one generation to the other, if they are lucky! This brings both much needed continuity to these businesses but also further grounds them within the daily business and social fabric of their communities.

If this connectedness to neighborhood is to continue to stay strong and even thrive, particularly invaluable in communities undergoing dramatic demographic changes, there are a variety of ways to accomplish this goal through the following actions requiring different levels of commitment (Tributetech.Com, 2022): (1) Serve on a community board; (2) Participate in community events; (3) Show your community what happens behind the scenes; (4) Share helpful content online; (5) Host events; and (6) Partner with other professionals.

These activities are found in other community-based organizations wishing to be further integrated into the daily activities of the people they serve in order to further an organization's mission. Further, these activities vary in type and intensity according to local circumstances, including the receptivity of the community to these overtures and the willingness and ability of funeral directors to carry them out in a respectful and faithful manner. When this harmony is interrupted, per the case of those owners facing danger themselves, it alters their future.

It would be a serious mistake to view funeral directors from a singular viewpoint because they perform multiple functions that often go unrecognized. Fletcher's (2022) interview with Karla Holloway (historian) regarding African-American funeral directors as preservers of culture and history is a perspective often overlooked in viewing the experiences resulting from trauma and deep pain, but with the potential to create resistance and resilience. Those in professional and academic circles, in turn, can seek meaningful involvement in shaping gun violence initiatives by purposefully reaching out to these establishments. Initiation of collaboration must not depend on one-side reaching out. Bridging this divide requires both sides venturing into unchartered terrain and developing partnerships with community needs guiding interventions.

This engagement cannot be imposed externally, requiring purposefully engaging them in the deliberation process with the goal of achieving trust. We must not forget it is their community and institutions. We, unless we live there, are guests. Community engagement (Andrade et al., 2021) is just not for the brave, reckless, and/or naïve, it is also for those who are wise and cautious among us in understanding our "guest" status. This concept highlights our precarious status and our potential to make welcome contributions.

One example of such an initiative is Philadelphia's collaboration between "Unity in the Community," a South Philadelphia afterschool program, and the Khadijah Alderman Funeral home. An afterschool carpentry program involving approximately a dozen students volunteering at least once a month at the funeral home. They undertake projects at the funeral home, such as building shelves and other activities hoping to break down barriers between this institution and the community they serve, in addition to better informing youth on the consequences of gun violence for themselves and their loved ones.

South Philadelphia is not the only neighborhood with community-initiated projects. These and other types of projects further integrate these establishments into the social fabric of their communities, increasing their influence and importance in the process. However, for projects to achieve any measure of success, they require meaningful involvement in crafting interventions. They must plan with rather than plan for them. This is not to say that there may not be suspicions of each other and walking on tender ground concerning the terms or vocabulary used, but the common denominator can be quite strong—namely, the health and wellbeing of residents/community.

Gun violence requires that social scientists and helping professions rethink how best to prevent and treat those injured and helping loved ones with emotional support (Delgado, 2022). The death care sector, particularly funeral services and cemeteries are a major segment of this field, and generally escaped scholarly attention in examining their role in addressing gun violence. The past decade witnessed this sector receiving increased attention, particularly from the popular press, both as providers and recipients of services due to their exposure to direct gun violence.

The Ever-Expanding Reach of Gun Violence-Related Grief

Defining the universe of a social problem is challenging and best left to those with the requisite nerves to do so. Doing so plays a significant role in shaping our analysis and response. A narrow definition severely limits responses, often simplifying what is a complex phenomenon; broadening the definition, in turn, necessitates being open to who is "worthy" of attention and resources. Gun trauma, too, comes in many different manifestations, as addressed in Chap. 4, challenging us in developing responses to match available resources and local circumstances (Abba-Aji et al., 2024). A "cookie-cutter" approach, as a result, is doomed to fail.

Models must bend to locales rather than the other way around. Readers with extensive urban practice experiences will not find this stance as strange. I like to say that planning is human and implementation is divine! When plans go as expected, it takes on a divine quality, without being disrespectful to readers who are religious. Grief is a profound universal human reaction we usually associate with losing loved ones or others close to us. It is critical that we eschew viewing grief as constituting a linear process, with corresponding stages. It is a dynamic process with progress and setbacks, which can be complicating by external events.

We do not know how the families of providers, too, are impacted by gun deaths. Teachers, for example, can grieve loss of their students; which, again we may not typically associate with grieving, particularly when these acts are violent and unexpected. We can take it a step further and identify fellow students who knew the victim and may have even been close friends (Gross, 2020, 2023, 2024), per Uvalde, and those outside of school (Beauplan, 2022). Human beings do not live in silos. Our lives are closely intertwined with the life of others. Research rarely extends its reach to these "other" individuals.

Readers can appreciate the vastness of the impact of a violent act on countless individuals and venues, many of whom may simply be invisible yet profoundly touched by violence. In extreme situations involving mass murders, the date this occurred may forever be marked as an anniversary, such as Sandy Hook and Uvalde, for example. Connecticut's Sandy Hook Elementary School was responsible for the nation having a visceral reaction to the mass killing of 6-year-olds, when on December 14, 2012, 20 children and two teachers were murdered in addition to leaving two injured, stunning the nation (Cherry, 2024). Grief can be channeled into social action, transforming into an act of social justice (Roland, 2021). It can also bring many different secondary gains, some totally unexpected. Nevertheless, there aren't enough of these exemplary examples to counteract the deleterious consequences of a gun.

The following description of one cemetery's special children's section is poignant, encapsulating the consequences of gun violence for families, loved ones, and those entrusted to bury them, including the emergence of a new way of thinking about cemeteries as "communities of the dead." These newfound communities, as per children lost to gun violence, have increasingly witnessed visitors who not only visit but also connect with others sharing similar experiences of having lost a child and developing a support system, bringing a trans-community view, too.

These special sections occupy an exalted "sanctuary" status. Catholic cemeteries, for example, often refer to these children's sections as "*Gardens of Angels*" or "*Holy Innocents'* Section," signifying the unique role they play. These sections will never be confused with the burials for any other group because they are easily identifiable by being adorned with statues and headstones characterizing the young ages of those buried there. These are sections set aside for "special" burials. Probably unexpectedly, also serving to connect visitors to each other for mutual support.

St. Louis, Missouri, too, has a cemetery ("Sunset Gardens of Memory") with a special children's section, bringing additional significance to those who work the grounds and help bury the dead, as in the case of Haire: "Haire says he's more than a groundskeeper, he's a caretaker. When a 3-year-old girl was shot and killed in the fall of 2021, Haire made sure she was buried in Baby Land. Haire started adding small touches to this part of the cemetery more than 30 years ago to make it feel special. He built a birdbath with angel statues that he painted by hand." Another groundskeeper touches on child burials (Anthony, 2023): "William Belt Sr., says it was awkward to walk by the gravestones without acknowledging them, so he greeted each one."

Those preparing the graves of young victims also have the responsibility to ensure that objects left at grave sites are well maintained. What do I mean by this? Latinos, for instance, have traditions of leaving objects at the sites of dead children, such as dolls (Calix & Denney-Koelsch, 2024). The graveyard of a little girl, for example, may have Barbie Dolls or other toys important to them, and effort is made to keep them the way they were laid out to honor family wishes. A birdbath may be left at a grave site because the child loved feeding birds and watching them bathe. These workers are also known to paint each angel in a children's section, including statues having the same skin pigmentation as the victims, which are often Black or Brown. Mind you, this artistry is not part of their job description!

Visitors, as noted throughout this book on where the Uvalde, Texas, child victims are buried, may be surprised to hear music, see dancing, and celebrations at the gravesites, almost as if the buried could still partake in a celebration of their birthdays, for example (Marketplace, 2024):

> From day one, these people that are affected by these profound, historic moments and by these tragedies are not avatars or symbols of grief or suffering. These are complex people with rich lives and relationships and senses of humor. And so, I feel that long-form storytelling is uniquely suited to help reveal some of those nuances. I think one photograph that sort of speaks to that is a photograph of Caitlyne Gonzales, who was in the classroom across the hall from the two classrooms where the shooting took place and many of her best friends were killed. She has become one of the youngest gun violence prevention advocates and she would often visit the cemetery to see her friends. She just went to her best friend Jackie's grave, and she took out her phone and started listening to Taylor Swift songs and listening to TikTok videos and dancing and being playful as if she was there with Jackie. And there was just something really profound and devastating about that, but also beautiful.

Contextualizing cemetery shootings helps us better understand the circumstances and nuances (indicators) that led to a shooting as well as assisting us in guarding against this violence through carefully researched and planned interventions. The roles groundkeepers play are obviously more than many of us would expect and cannot be overlooked in this search for new knowledge and interventions. No aspect of this job is perfunctory, including its ramifications on those in this sector. Children's sections are expanding across the nation, although I could not gather statistics on this movement. This illustration is reflective of the increasing numbers of children dying by gun violence, a key dimension to this public health problem. In 2023, Philadelphia, Pennsylvania, for example, experienced a 24-hour shooting period with victims, including the youngest victim 2-year-old killed in his crib (Philadelphia Inquirer, 2024).

The ages of young victims necessitates that their burials occupy a special status in varied ways, differentiating them from other burials, eschewing a "business as usual" approach to how and where they are buried. These special considerations include those entrusted to care for these plots. This violent act ascends to even greater significance because it involves young children in what should be considered a safe space as symbolized by an elementary school. Further, cemeteries can set aside a special children's section (Anthony, 2023):

> 'This is 'Baby Land,' said Haire, Sunset Gardens' grounds supervisor, as he gestured across the area. 'This is where a lot of babies are buried.' Cemeteries like this one have long honored those who die too young. Such special burial sites exist ... They are for stillborn children and those who died of disease or accidents. Today, a modern epidemic fills more graves than anything else: In the U.S., firearm-related injuries were the leading cause of death for children in 2020, ahead of motor vehicle crashes ... The men at Sunset Gardens are collecting data in their own way, too. In 2019, Haire broke ground on a new section ... where teenagers and young adults are buried, including those killed by COVID-19 and many who were victims of gun violence. It's called the 'Garden of Grace.' It's already been used more than anyone would like... The groundskeepers at Sunset Gardens have learned to watch their step in Baby Land because grieving parents drop off toys, candy, and balloons for their deceased children. 'They just do things so differently in grief ...

A "special cemetery children's section" may be new to many readers. It is a manifestation of the special circumstances surrounding their death and final resting place. Further, when their deaths are disproportionately due to guns, it speaks to our inability or unwillingness as a society to address this public health problem in this nation's cities. If we, as a nation, can tolerate children being killed, then no group is immune.

All gun deaths are very sad, tragic, and often unexpected, bringing long-term anticipated and unanticipated consequences, more so for young children, even in a high gun violence environment. "Special burials," such as those involving young children, are not business as usual for the death care sector. Their numbers are increasingly calling for special initiatives to aid loved ones and those called on to carry out their work responsibilities when they go home at the end of the day (Anthony, 2023):

> 'I weep,' he said. 'Big difference between crying and weeping. Weeping, I'm closer to God.' Their job is physical, emotional work done in all seasons, all weather. Injuries occur. Heartbreak is everywhere. To hold their own hearts together, the groundskeepers often decompress as they eat lunch in a shed near the cemetery's front office, trading stories in front of a wood-burning stove to keep warm during winter. They find joy where they can. The Belts like to fish. And the senior Belt occasionally sings the blues to soothe his soul... And they laugh when they can. William Belt Sr. still remembers his first year on the job. He wanted to be respectful, he said with a smile, even though his clients were deceased. These type of burial takes an extraordinary toll on those who work in this sector:

Child burials stand out for their emotional toll on funeral workers (https://www.youtube.com/watch?v=noEAg0sMnMc). One does not have to be a parent to have an intense emotional upheaval that these deaths cause. Interventions must be sufficiently flexible (dynamic) to take this and other considerations into the approaches taken, allowing community circumstances and history to weigh in on the final outcome. This chapter's illustrations introduced a new arena for urban gun practice, undertaking research, and broadening gun violence practice in service to the families and communities of these victims.

Cemetery workers do not hold positions that are highly paid, prestigious, or glamorous for young children to aspire to become upon growing up. In other words, they are not role models or high-profile positions to hold from a community or society standpoint. In many ways, cemetery workers are invisible. This may in part be the result of the circumstances and the pain of those attending these last rites. That status does not take away from their importance, particularly during crisis periods caused by gun violence.

Unlike other roles portrayed in the media, there are no television shows or movies depicting them, their challenges, and the vital roles they play in communities and society; they have no faces, feelings, histories, or experiences, so to speak. There are never portrayed as heroes even when their actions during gun violence incidents save lives. Not having a face or name translates into being a non-entity. When attending a burial, we are not in our most observant selves and the event takes on more of a blur, which makes sense from a personal standpoint. We think of the death care sector only when we have to or unless something dramatic happens there that makes local news. Ironically, it is a sector that we can never avoid.

Their invisibility also applies to their pain. This means that in carrying out their responsibilities, they pay an immense price to their emotional health, including their physical well-being when they are caught-up in the line of fire. Their families, too, must contend with the fallout of this violence and corresponding intense emotions. Where do they turn to for much needed support? These workers provide a valuable community service that must be recognized and supported.

The Robb Elementary School, Uvalde, Texas (2022), mass shooting, as noted earlier, made national and international news because of the horrific nature of this violent act on young children and their teachers, raising serious questions about live shooting protocols and police force actions. There is a common saying among gun advocates that a "good guy" with a gun trumps a "bad guy with a gun." There were well over 100 police officers at the scene, all carrying guns, and that did not stop the carnage that transpired over an extended period of time while the police were present! Those circumstances made a tragic situation even worse for this community and victim families, because countless children could have been saved but were not because of inaction or mis-action, and not to mention the town itself.

Uvalde's children caskets were not the typical caskets one associates with gun killings, and I venture to guess that this aspect of the funeral scene is new to most readers. Its frequency, at the very least, is alarming. Child burials bring considerations different from their adult counterparts. First of all, the sizes of these caskets make it difficult to obtain because young children cannot be buried in an adult casket. Further, efforts to individualize a death are certainly not new, as evidenced by the objects left in a casket. The emergence of "casket wraps," for example, allow parents to individually decorate their children's caskets, illustrating how children bring special challenges and opportunities (Kai, 2022).

> With mass shootings becoming the *leading cause of death* for children in the United States since 2020, the *need for child-sized coffins* has grown at a similarly alarming rate. However, only one manufacturer in the nation makes them. *Cherokee Child Caskets in Griffin, Ga.* is on its own when it comes to providing families in the United States with final resting places specifically designed for children. Since 1941, Cherokee has provided over 10,000 different child caskets and products that vary in size, color, styles, and other personalized options ... More than a decoration, the wraps for the children in Uvalde are intended to offer solace in time of devastation and serve as reminders that the problem of gun violence remains unresolved. Whether wrapped in an image, decoration, memorabilia, or something else, mourners are discovering meaningful ways to say farewell to loved ones. *Damian Ferek*, president of the West Virginia company, explained to *Kaiser Health News* that wraps often incorporate superheroes and rainbows, unicorns and teddy bears, alongside photos of the smiling children.

Grief is an overwhelming human emotion, especially after experiencing a trauma, such as losing a child, and particularly to gun violence. Finding ways to help them cope with this tragedy is critical. For many, art is a coping mechanism, such as decorating wraps. Families often see more than just a casket but as a source of joy for their child, helping parents and loved ones feel closer to their deceased children. It is a small, yet sometimes a powerful way to assist families with the emotional onus of burying a child and mourning their loss.

Hillcrest Memorial Cemetery's children's section has not returned to business as usual because of this tragic shooting. It altered what can be considered sacred ground in a profound manner. Again, not surprisingly, it ascended to occupy an exalted and critical position of helping these families and their community in their moment of grief (Kalifa, 2023):

> The families of the *21 people* who were killed have spent the last year working their way through a wilderness of grief, anger, despair, frustration and confusion — searching, if not for peace, then at least purpose. The cemetery, where most of the victims are buried, has become an anchor for many of the families, as has the bond forged among them. The families decorate the graves and meticulously maintain the area surrounding the headstones; and together, they gather at the cemetery to celebrate birthdays and holidays.

A cemetery is much more than a piece of land, a serene setting, a place for burials and last rites to be administered, and a place and space for loved ones to visit and pay respects. In other words, "an eternal resting place" with the emphasis on resting. That is not hard to fathom when we think of these places and spaces from a traditional viewpoint. Cemeteries are often called sacred lands, places, and spaces. Cemeteries are also a form of libraries of the dead as keepers of stories harboring repositories of memories for families, highlighting a high level of significance for them and their communities. We must not forget that cemeteries are communal spaces.

The circumstances of the Uvalde children's deaths, including the two teachers also killed, have assumed added symbolic meaning, even ascending to a status as a sanctuary, in the truest sense of the word. In gist, it has joined the community they serve in a way that many of us, including this author, would not have thought possible. This cemetery became an extension for families and their community, highly unusual for cemeteries, as discussed later in this book. We usually think of cemeteries as separate spaces and places. That separation, as a result, may not exist in some communities. Cemeteries bring much needed spaces that can accommodate large groups to mourn communally.

Cemetery workers, in turn, experience emotional burdens when witnessing and supporting these families. Where do they receive support in helping them deal with this traumatic event? Obviously, they need resources that consider their unique circumstances. Unfortunately, options are limited, unless they are lucky enough to have a supervisor able to take on this responsibility, either personally or obtaining outside support. This may include enlisting outside help when an emergency occurs, considering this act as part of their job description and employee benefit. Having instrumental or expressive support available to these workers is not an extraordinary request in high gun violence contexts.

The healthcare sector, too, occupies a prominent position in the death care industry if we venture outside of a small circle of institutions and individuals tasked with burials. Nurses, for example, need support due to their healthcare roles and how they are often called on to engage parents and other loved ones about the death of a relative/patient (Reny et al., 2020). Social workers, too, can be tasked to follow-up in providing counseling and connecting the bereaved to resources and connecting with the death care sector.

It may be surprising that death's place in a medical curriculum is considered deficient (Dombroski, 2023), calling for introducing this content into a crowded curriculum. Anyone who has developed curriculum will acknowledge the dilemma that brings as to what content to include or exclude. Sadly, those in medical education have much to learn about dying and death (Rosenblatt & Wallace, 2021). Other helping professions, too, can share a similar conclusion. Television shows often have doctors fulfilling this role before running off to deal with another patient or a medical emergency. Nevertheless, that is not always the case. This is not to say any profession has an easy task addressing this trauma. However, what support do nurses and doctors receive to aid them if sought out, for example? If so, that is very helpful; if not, it brings a trauma onus for them and their loved ones (Hodder, 2024).

How notification of a traumatic death is conveyed to loved ones, for example, and not surprisingly, must embrace the challenges that this act entails, which are multifaceted and take into account local circumstances (McCarroll et al., 2024):

> when survivors elect to and are permitted to see the body, every effort should be made by those responsible for the body to assure that the survivors are: (a) prepared for what they will see and may experience; (b) given a private location and time in which to reflect on the challenges that they face; (c) provided answers to all questions by authorities who have knowledge of the circumstances of the death; (d) permitted to perform rituals according to their faith and culture, within reason and with an appreciation of the limitations of where the body is viewed and (e) given a follow-up call with a staff professional such as a nurse or social worker after they leave the facility in order to answer any remaining questions and provide support and resources, if desired.

These responsibilities do not rest with one individual, setting, or time, and those in the death care sector will find themselves in this system of delivery for the bereaved. Grief does not lend itself to being limited to one setting or time period since it is an emotion that can get exacerbated by certain geographical settings and over a course of time. That complicates how we view and treat it when it escalates in severity and it interferes with daily functioning.

Readers may think that professionally trained providers that address gun trauma will automatically be able to personally deal with the consequences of this violence and have the necessary ongoing supervisory support when needed. That is not always the case, it bears noting (Semenza & Kravitz-Wirtz, 2024). Those whose experience has been positive in this realm, please be assured that you are very fortunate. Even professionals harden by daily urban violence experiences cannot escape its profound emotional toll as described by Dr. Simons (2023):

> I've experienced firsthand how the story of one bullet's devastation goes way beyond what we see in the ED as our football team, high school, and community grieved for Tyce over the past week. I listened to a fellow football mom wail beside her son's casket. I heard sniffles from nearly every person in a church filled to standing room only. I watched tears stream down countless cheeks as one of the friends with Tyce when he was shot spoke from the pulpit about what he said as they drove him to the hospital. 'He was saying that he just wanted to see his mom and dad and brother again.' I have a hard time seeing someone mortally wounded die in front of me, and I'm trained for it. I felt for this poor kid who watched his friend die. His psyche will be one of the many secondary casualties of the bullet that killed Tyce.

We must be reminded that this testimonial is made by an emergency room physician, who in the course of a workday encounters patients in dire circumstances and should be "battle hardened" by their training and experiences. Nevertheless, one can ask the question can anyone ever really forget such an event at the end of the day? Imagine the mental health field simply ignoring that they exist? That is what can be said for those in the death care sector. Hospital staff in urban communities must contend with high volumes of patients with life and death gun injuries and the corresponding trauma they must live with as they struggle to save lives and when they fail, having to inform loved ones who were clinging to hope (Miller, 2023):

> Seeing so many cases of needless gun violence takes a toll. Depression, PTSD, and anxiety can all emerge from repeatedly treating victims and having hard conversations with their families. Quickly moving on to the next patient *feels empty of empathy yet is expected.* Hospital staff are *struggling more than ever* and repeated instances of gun violence can be triggering— especially for Black staff who feel the extra burden of racialized gun and police violence. Black hospital workers may feel the impacts even deeper when working with Black victims. It's traumatizing to try and save a gun or police violence victim with the knowledge that you personally belong to the group being targeted.

I cannot imagine someone dealing with the immense consequences of gun violence without this training and professional support usually provided through supervision, in-service training, or consultation, for example. They cannot simply turn off the images and stories of someone killed by an assault rifle when they go off-duty! When this happens to a young child, the image can stay for a lifetime. The concept of co-victim comes to mind, with implications for their social network, too, contending with these emotional consequences and ill equipped to do so. This concept will reappear due to its saliency in understanding how it impacts segments of a community, including the deathcare sector.

The funeral business plays an instrumental role in our society and it is complex. It must respond to local circumstances in order to remain relevant. Unfortunately, that means that the method of death, as in the case of gun violence, must now come front and center in urban high gun violence communities for the safety of personnel and consumers.

Urban Gangs: An Overview

One cannot author a book on urban gun violence without acknowledging gangs and the significant and destructive (instrumental and expressive) role that they play in causing this public health problem. Any word association of the term "gang" elicits a variety of negative names and images, including gun violence, because of their prominence on television shows and movies. This country has a vivid and distressing image of gangs, with corresponding reactions to them, mostly negative and fearful. If one were to play word association with gangs, it would not be surprising to see high-powered guns, violence, fighting, pain, sorrow, drugs, extortion, and deaths prominently on most readers' list. This list would be universal regardless of our location in the country, and I would venture to say, internationally, too.

It is important to provide at least a simple definition of what constitutes a "gang." A gang, according to the United States Department of Justice, is an explicitly formed association consisting of at least three individuals with the expressed intent of creating terror or seeking to intimate other groups (Garcia-Rojo et al., 2023). Readers wishing an erudite definition will not have difficulty finding it on this subject. The naming of a gang, in turn, is not a haphazard process when utilizing framing theory, and much thought is devoted to this activity (Kearley et al., 2024).

Urban gangs play a prominent role in creating and shaping an atmosphere of fear of community gun violence (Ceccato & Westman, 2024; Urban Institute, 2018). The concept of the lone gunmen, for example, rarely exists in high gun violence communities. However, gang gun violence seems to dominate the field of pain and sorrow. Readers may associate gang membership with a plethora of risky behaviors. Interestingly, gangs are often overlooked as a key source of urban mortality among youth (Pyrooz et al., 2020). Arresting gang leaders, for example, has shown that it can reduce gun violence (Burke, 2024), but not solve the problem because it shows the pervasiveness of the problem.

An in-depth coverage of gangs is beyond this book's scope, although it would be irresponsible to ignore them due to their prominence in mass shootings and murders during last rites at sacred sites. This illustrates that no space, time, and place is beyond the reach of this violence. Gang research and interventions are a significant sub-field of criminology for very good reasons because they bring unique qualities and influences on community well-being and dynamics.

Individuals without gang affiliations perpetrate gun violence at key moments at last rite ceremonies, too. Nevertheless, there will invariably be a gang connection at the root of this violence. Solving the problem of urban gangs goes a long way toward addressing, or at least seriously mitigating, the problem of gun violence. Urban gangs are a part of urban history, which we must not forget (Howell, 2015). Gangs wield tremendous influence on their communities in multiple ways as touched upon in this book.

Bruhn (2021), for example, found that Chicago gangs reduce median property values an average of $8436.9 and household income $1866.80 where present. These are considerable sums in low-income communities on a subject most readers, I would venture to guess, have not considered. Gangs, we must not forget, distort funds from local businesses, compromising their "bottom-line" and discouraging other businesses from locating in these neighborhoods internationally and nationally (Neu, 2023). These costs, in turn, are passed on to customers, who are often ill-prepared to pay them without sacrifice.

Gangs are increasingly recognized by urban communities and law enforcement as a key force in increasing violence and more specifically shootings, although there are other entities that must not be ignored because of their importance. Urban gangs are a subset within the criminology field due to their significance in shaping crime and more specifically violence.

This section covers five aspects of urban gun violence, providing parameters for viewing their role and significance in shaping this violence: (1) Importance of Collective Group Identity; (2) Gangs as Protection; (3) Collective Violence; (4) The Evolution of Gang Violence; and (5) Gangbanging at Funerals. These arenas overlap, although often treated as separate sections.

Importance of Collective Group Identity

The concept of identity is well recognized by scholars, practitioners, and ordinary people on the street due to its importance in shaping how we view ourselves and others. Collective group identity, in turn, is central to gang existence, including how they name themselves. Lauger (2020) argues that collective group identity has been neglected in the gang literature where a name captures an identity and belonging is such a powerful force. Growing up in the South Bronx, it was a fact that gangs existed, were violent, and with reputations taking on a greater than life status, touching every resident in one form or another.

This topic is personal. Further, there was never any question on the boundaries of their "territories" and the importance of avoiding these spaces or "spots" if possible. That made it more difficult to go to school, for example, because we could not follow the shortest path to get there. "Navigation" took on new meaning, and not just for getting to and from school (Barboza-Salerno & Meshelemiah, 2023). That experience stays with you for a lifetime. Although the concept of identity has received substantial attention from sociologists and psychologists, it has not been well developed in the gang literature.

Violence's varied manifestation, particularly when involving guns, is instrumental in gang identity due to its association with strength/power. Violence was central in their origins and maintaining self-respect. It served a symbolic role (street reputation) in the creation of collective identity, in addition to serving instrumental ends by generating economic enterprises, such as extortion (Neu, 2023), which often constituted "protection" to local businesses, for example, and drug activity (Valasik & Reid, 2021). Gang members must have their basic needs met to continue to exist and attract new members (Sonterblum, 2018).

Fear of violence is a key mechanism gangs rely on to maintain social control. Gangs are usually characterized by their willingness to exercise violence (Ibrahim et al., 2024). The saying "all bark and no bite" helps describe a gang unwilling to exercise violence. Pointing to high visibility victims as examples reinforces this attempt at control and the futility of challenging it. No one is safe and no situation is off-limits to exercising this power. Gang violence, using guns and/or destroying or disrespecting graves, is such an example, as seen in the case illustrations of Boston and Jacksonville in this book. This is a formula for violence without concerns for the ultimate victims, such as that experienced in the death care sector.

Gang violence, too, has evolved with easier access to guns, particularly assault-type weapons, introducing a new and deadly dimension to the reign of terror that they bring to communities. The more powerful weapons a gang possesses and their willingness to use them, the stronger they are perceived as being and the greater their potential destructive power. Possessing these weapons without using them does little to quell community concerns. Use of these weapons is essential to display power.

Social media as a communication tool has changed, making it easier for gang members to communicate with each other, playing a critical role in fostering gun violence (Szabo, 2023):

> Juan Campos has been working to save at-risk teens from gun violence for 16 years. As a street outreach worker in Oakland, California, he has seen the pull and power of gangs... But, he said, he's never confronted a force as formidable as social media, where small boasts and disputes online can escalate into deadly violence in schoolyards and on street corners. Teens post photos or videos of themselves with guns and stacks of cash, sometimes calling out rivals, on Facebook, Instagram, Snapchat, or TikTok. When messages go viral, fueled by 'likes' and comments, the danger is hard to contain, Campos said.

This communication enhancement sets the stage for gun violence by facilitating coordination during death ceremonies as a means of retribution and gang reputation maintenance and/or enhancement. These attacks are often well planned, particularly when there is a total disregard for collateral damage, guaranteeing that the message of "don't defy" us gets out. Life, in essence, becomes "cheap" and therefore expendable.

Gangs as Protection

Deadly violence's pervasiveness, often due to gangs and guns, needs no further coverage here because it permeates this entire book. Ironically, joining a gang is often motivated by someone attempting to obtain protection from violence and life's structural inequalities, yet it further exposes members to potentially deadly violence (Swaner, 2022), including family members. If members are killed by a rival gang, they can expect to be revenged. This is a small consolation to being murdered. Nevertheless, their death will extract a heavy price in return, hoping to serve as a deterrence, although a very weak one from my standpoint.

A "Catch 22" emerges in gang member lives exposing them to an increased likelihood of imprisonment (De Vito, 2020) and personal dangers, and their family, too, when they are killed and violence continues as they are put to rest. Joining a gang translates into families being considered "fair territory" for revenge violence regardless of their backgrounds, with children and youth being at the wrong place and time when this occurs. It is almost as if one family member joins a gang, an entire family joins, too. Funeral homes, houses of worship, and graveside shootings will invariably have revenge at the center of the dispute, and can be defined as "perceived harm to one's wellbeing" as a key motivator (DiBlasi & Kassinove, 2022, p. 873).

When a family member joins a gang, the probability of a sibling joining increases. So-called "cracks in the family" make it easier to find instrumental and expressive needs being met in gangs (Assari et al., 2020). I remember talking with a gang member that had a sibling in the same gang. He said "I have two families. One I was born into and the other I joined with my brother." Readers new to communities with high levels of gang participation may have trouble understanding this point. This also helps explain gun violence at burials. Gang members have a functional family (gang) and a biological family, with instances where these forms of family become one, blurring the lines between these two worlds (De Vito, 2020; Hashimi et al., 2021). When a gang member leaves, they become stigmatized, much in similar fashion to having a family member outcasted (Lee & Bubolz, 2020).

Collective Violence

Violence needs viewing from a variety of lens, including a collective vision. We must keep an open mind on what is a violent act, including what constitutes a collective act, bringing high visibility. Krug et al.'s (2002, p. 213) definition of collective violence helps us view gang violence—"the instrumental use of violence by people who identify themselves as members of a group—whether this group is transitory or has a more permanent identity—against group or set of individuals, in order to achieve political, economic, or social objectives."

This definition emphasizes violence in achieving instrumental (concrete) and expressive (psychological) goals not limited to gangs but clearly embraced by gangs. We must not forget that gangs are not "friendship groups." Expressive goals encompass a variety of acts such as when violence occurs during a death ceremony. The victim being buried cannot die again. However, that victim is not the "real" target of this violence, as seen in the case illustrations where gravestones are destroyed or social media is used to disrespect a deceased gang member. Rather, the intent is to send a public message to a broader audience at the ceremony. The central purpose of the threat is collective rather than aimed at an individual.

The Evolution of Gang Violence from Rumbles to Gang Bangers and Drive-Bys

It is worth providing an overview of how gang violence has evolved over the past several decades, including changing the burial scene in the process. Gangs have been part of this nation's history with urbanization of the late nineteenth century witnessing tremendous growth in their numbers and lethality with the availability of guns. Sander's book *Gangbangs and drive-bys: Grounded culture and juvenile gang violence* captures the evolution of gang violence from its origins as "rumbles," a term from the 1950s and 1960s. Manufactured guns replaced knives, switchblades, bats, and heavy chains as weapons of choice. The days of hand-to-hand combat are relegated to history with guns altering the modern-day battlefield.

The term "gang bangers" is often used to describe gang members using guns to perpetrate violence. Any and all deaths due to gang violence can be considered a tragedy with associated sorrow and misery. These deaths are hardly ever "natural" or the result of "old age" of one long retired. However, within the constellation of deaths, there is a hierarchy with children at the top of this list. Who is at the bottom? Those engaging in gun violence as a way of life, regardless of the circumstances that led to their demise, probably occupy this position.

The term gang banger captures an image of this individual, with a string of violent and reckless acts, which can also include taking someone's life as an initiation ceremony. When one of them dies because of gun violence, it brings sorrow for their family, but it also places a community on "edge" because the ramifications of this death can cause additional deaths and pain, creating a vicious cycle of retaliation causing greater misery throughout a neighborhood. Fellow gang members will often seek to have a memorable sendoff to them.

Calling killings of gang members as "deaths of despair" helps humanize them (Aspholm, 2022) in a world where pain and suffering are prosaic, and they, in turn, play a key role in this despair. Gang members in the constellation of gun victims will probably not stand out in any hierarchy of victims from a community standpoint. That does not mean that there are not loved ones and others who are severely saddened by their death. These loved ones must rely on each other for solace and comfort. When gun violence occurs during a ceremony where they are saying their final goodbyes, they, too, must seek and obtain solace and comfort from others.

The stressors and structural barriers youth of color face are immense and well documented (Tyson McCrea et al., 2024). Gun violence takes center stage in their lives because of the lethality of weapons. Nevertheless, at the very least, these other stressors interfere with "healthy" living and healing. The quest for a "good funeral," and I would add "safe," is a goal for this industry (Long & Lynch, 2013), and for families and other loved ones of the deceased. This goal, nevertheless, needs grounding from practical, cultural, and symbolic standpoints. A "cookie-cutter" approach is doomed to fail by not meeting the varied needs of attendees at a last rites ceremony, particularly in highly diverse urban communities.

There are significant efforts across other urban centers where houses of worship have undertaken gun violence initiatives or engaged in coalitions, as illustrated in the following examples. In Baltimore, a buy-back program was initiated by a local church rather than a non-profit (U.S. Catholics, 2024):

> On a hot summer morning last August, a long line of cars waited in the Edmondson Village Shopping Center in Baltimore. The drivers, including some who arrived two hours early, were there to exchange weapons for money, no questions asked, during a gun buyback event organized by the nearby St. Joseph Monastery Parish. Father Mike Murphy ... was inspired to organize the buyback because of his city's ongoing struggles with gun violence. From 2015 to 2022, his city surpassed a devastating 300 homicides per year. Murphy chose the shopping center location because a young man had been killed there earlier in the year while on a lunch break from his school. 'Our goal was to get weapons off the street as much as possible,' Murphy says. 'Having it in a place where somebody lost his life was a way of showing, 'We have to do better at promoting a culture of peace.' Murphy worked with diocesan partners to raise $60,000 for the event, which paid $200 to 300 per gun ... the team collected 362 weapons to melt down, including 17 semi-automatic weapons and three guns that had been previously reported stolen.

This example is one of countless others carried out nationally for houses of worship to aid a community struggling with gun violence. Having churches join in the fight on guns brings them into closer contact with potential dangers and the fight for control of territories within neighborhoods. When houses of worship upset the status quo they face, the wrath of those in power viewing this institution as a threat. These efforts endear these institutions while concomitantly presenting challenges to local gangs and others wishing to maintain the status quo. Any student of history will see how houses of worship have found themselves in deadly power struggles with governments threatened by its power.

We must not be surprised that the reach of inequities finds its way into trauma care. Inequities do not just start at a trauma center. The relationship of transport time to a trauma center and death after a gunshot wound is a dimension of care we may not typically think of when discussing this form of medical service. Victims of color, compared to White, non-Latinos, had significantly longer transport times to trauma centers and predicted mortality would have been lower with White victim transport times. Stop the Bleed campaigns, discussed elsewhere in this book, must be offered in high gun violence communities.

Gang Violence at Funerals

This is a good point to spotlight gun violence at houses of worship, which will be addressed in greater depth throughout the remaining sections of this book, particularly in Chap. 7 on Pittsburgh, Pennsylvania. Funeral gang violence is not new but its frequency and deadly outcomes have caused increased attention due to the consequences it brings to communities and the challenges it presents in stopping it during ceremonies (FuneralWise, in press):

> It is a painful irony that funerals can promote violence and instill fear in family members and friends... gang funerals follow the traditions of the deceased's religious or cultural affiliations. Whether they are AME (African Methodist Episcopal) or New Orleans Jazz funerals, the specifics are left up to the family and the deceased's wishes. In some cases, families, friends, and members of the community seize the opportunity of the funeral to plead with gang members to stop the violence and promote peace in the streets... Rival gang members often seek retribution or threaten violence against family and friends at funerals. Sometimes it is simply a way that gangs can intimidate each other... In 1990, five people were shot in Linden, N.J. Men posing as funeral mourners ditched their floral bouquets and fired machine guns and a shotgun into a crowd of 100 people... Panic broke out at the sound of gunfire, and several of the mourners in attendance were injured. Because of the risks associated with gang violence, funerals of gang members are likely to be avoided by members of the community out of fear.

I imagine that most readers are familiar with New Orlean's Second-line parades where collective mourning transforms into collective joy (Sakakeeny, 2024). Hunter (2024) draws attention to the role and importance of second-line parades as a trauma-informed response by families and communities to grief. Introducing gun violence to this solemn occasion integrates music, celebration, and tradition as a backdrop.

An inability for grieving families and other loved ones to surround themselves with others sharing their sorrows is a dimension that again, because of how we typically think of gun violence, is simply overlooked in any statistical accounting. Specificity of setting (socio-cultural) for gun violence is essential in a comprehensive accounting of the public spaces and places where it occurs. This also calls for a qualitative and quantitative picture to emerge, with lessons to be learned on how communities can come together to mourn, although recognizing that New Orleans, Louisiana, brings a unique history of Afro-Creole and African-American New Orleanians to these celebrations (Carrico, 2024).

Urban gangs, as covered in this section, are a prominent fixture in any attempt at understanding gun violence and the death care sector, taking into account regional considerations as evidenced in the New Orleans case example covered above. The richness of final rites allows final rites to be customized to account for the background of the victims being honored.

Death Care PTSD

There are numerous invisible consequences that manifest themselves in the gun violence field. Urban gun trauma is not limited to family members of the deceased but has also spilled over to the death care scene (Moselle, 2021): "Arranging more funerals for gunshot victims has also made Forrest's business more dangerous. He says there's always the possibility of someone showing up at a church or a cemetery to fire off a few shots, particularly if the murder was committed by a member of a rival street group." The more cynical observer may argue that gun violence is good for business, so why are those in the funeral sector complaining? There are many natural causes to continue to provide enough "business" and this industry does not need gun violence to remain viable.

Adu et al. (2023) argue that mortuary workers can change their practices in response to changing circumstance, as per deaths due to COVID; however, families are generally resistant to these changes. Their research, based in Indonesia, but the results resonate with my experiences in the United States. Changing long-held culturally expected rituals because of gun violence fears will cause loved ones to react in the same manner, making policy changes in how funerals are conducted that are much more challenging to achieve.

Death care staff (funeral directors or undertakers, which are sometimes referred to as mortuary workers) do suffer from PTSD but have been ignored as a sub-group for specialized help. We may question how difficult has the work of morticians gotten? Chan (2022) offers a rare glimpse into this world and the challenges they face with assault-style weapons increasingly making their work more arduous, as evident in the following description of their work:

> Not much stuns mortician Hari Close after embalming more than 12,000 bodies over 30 years. But Close was left speechless last spring when he was tasked with preparing the body of a man who had been shot in the head with an assault-style weapon. Close worked alone

> in his funeral home in Baltimore for 26 h over three days, hoping plaster, clay and other materials could give the man's family the closure that comes with an open-casket funeral. But there was not much he could do. The top half of the man's head was gone. 'Imagine a full face, cut in half. It looked like half of an egg,' Close said. 'There was nothing there.'

One does not go home at the end of a shift after a horrific shooting without nightmares about this experience. Funeral attendees cannot view the body of their loved ones as it is customarily done, making the final services that much more painful. There is a good reason why the term "weapons of war" exists. They are not meant to wound but to destroy a human body and demoralize the "enemy."

McClanahan (2020), in a rare study on posttraumatic stress among mortuary workers, found that urban female workers displayed a propensity for higher PTSD scores when compared to male counterparts in rural settings. Urban workers, in turn, experienced higher PTSD scores compared to rural counterparts. The stigma of serving the lower-class, too, introduces classism to the factors associated with PTSD. McClanahan (2020, p. 7) notes that identification with the deceased is also operative in the life of these workers: "Identification with the deceased is a cognitive mechanism in which someone who works with the dead experiences feelings such as 'It could have been me,' 'It could have been my spouse,' or 'It could have been my friend.'"

Protective factors may counter negative forces such as compassion satisfaction and coping skills. This is particularly so when workers share many of the sociodemographic characteristics as the deceased. In cases where the mental health consequences are severe, professional stigma wields great influence in seeking much needed help more difficult.

Gun deaths also made a difficult job more physically demanding and emotionally draining. This form of death is also associated with anticipatory stress, particularly among new workers and female staff members. According to the U.S. Department of Health and Human Services (2020): "Mortuary and death care workers routinely come into contact with death and human remains as part of their professional roles. As a result, resiliency is built through experience, education, and peer support. However, for many working in this profession it may be uncommon to discuss or reveal their emotions and perceived stress to others."

Readers wishing to further read stories of surviving victims dealing with the profound challenges in the aftermath of gun violence are recommended to read Bates' (2024) book *In These Streets: Reporting from the Front Lines of Inner-City Gun Violence.* This book draws on extensive interviews and stories of victims, perpetrators, community activists, and academics, in bringing a multifaceted perspective on urban gun violence and efforts to prevent this violence and helping victims heal. Even though it is a prosaic problem in many cities, no two stories are similar. We must not neglect this pool of talent in helping communities start their journey of recovery. There is greater attention being paid to gun violence staff and job-related trauma exposure after an extended period where this topic escaped popular and scholarly attention; this neglect causes them severe strains in their personal lives and even situations where they turned to mind-altering substances and high-risk behaviors (Free & MacDonald, 2022).

A rare study of funeral worker health and safety, although based in Australia and Ireland but with implications for the United States, found work-related stress, fatigue from manually handling human remains, and exposure to biological hazards (Roche et al., 2022), with children often presenting the greatest challenges for these workers, as found in the United States:

> Working with the bereaved and the dead imposed emotional demands. All participants reported funerals for children or following violent deaths as the most emotionally challenging role aspects: 'Two days after Christmas and they're only one day old, your head doesn't even know how to deal with that. You get all depressed. They're the ones that really, really, mess with the head ... I did the funeral for that child, and that is possibly the single most uncomfortable thing I've done in my life … Then I went and had a breakdown afterwards.' (pp. 9–10)

Although this study is based in countries not known for gun violence, the findings were not surprising, and I have found them to be applicable to experiences in this country. This industry cannot continue to be ignored by the violence prevention and treatment field, with gun violence, not appliable in the above example, still weighing heavily.

Gang Burials and Gun Violence

The subjects of urban gangs, violence, and burials will not elicit any surprise from urban practitioners. High gun presence often equates with high gang violence, including deaths. Gang-related shootings as a subset of urban shootings are beyond the scope of this book, although considerable attention on various aspects of gang violence will be devoted to this topic. I cannot author this book without attention to urban gangs, although it is unfair to lay this problem solely at the doorsteps of gangs. Individual, non-gang affiliated gun violence is also a reality.

Gun carrying for self-protection is salient in high violence communities. Historically, there is a recognition that identifying and intervening with first-time gun carrying is a critical stage in preventing gun violence in low resource urban communities. The consequences of early onset of gun carrying result in a higher likelihood of engaging in violence (Dong & Wilson, 2024). Possessing a gun by Black-Americans may have more to do with self-protection (Comer & Connolly, 2020) rather than intending to perpetrate an act of aggression, per Baltimore, Maryland; Jackson, Mississippi; Houston, Texas; and Wilmington, Delaware study (Dillard et al., 2023, p. 197): "As our findings highlight, the environment exposes young Black men to guns and gun violence at an early age. The exposure to violence frequently puts them in a position in which gun possession is necessary." Having more guns does not translate into safer communities, however.

This book has not addressed how an increase in gun availability translates into higher rates of suicide, for example. Research on gun violence exposure (hearing gunshots near home or the slaying of friends or classmates) among Black-American adults aged 18–94 is linked to higher suicide risk; 12% of the study's sample experienced three or more gun violence exposures. New research shows cumulative effects (The Guardian, 2024): "'In the hood, you don't discuss being scared,' Bari, now 49, said. 'But as a youngster, you're consumed with these thoughts at all times. You're playing these scenarios in your head day to day. Mentally, you're a wreck.'" Countering exposure to neighborhood violence and gun carrying among adolescents is best countered when they have the benefit of protective parents, highlighting the importance of having parents present (Baiden et al., 2024).

These shootings, particularly when causing high numbers of injuries rather than deaths, are arduous to clear from a judicial standpoint (Barao et al., 2021). Fears of retribution are at the heart of reluctance to cooperate with law enforcement. This culture creates a sense of impunity, further increasing the likelihood that violence can be committed and justice does not prevail in the conventional sense. "Street justice," also called "cultural honor" (Whaley, 2022), comes through a violent act of equal or greater consequences in return, creating a vicious cycle with an ever-ending string of victims along the way.

Further, gang shootings are more lethal than non-gang shootings (Brantingham et al., 2021). Thus, the death care sector is put on notice to expect more burials of gang members and lethal violence to increase. This can carry over to death ceremonies and potentially compromising other burials and the institutions involved in this final act. The spillover consequences of these acts of violence are simply the cost of doing business. This is such a sad statement to make because of how it causes many lives being cut short, and for those who "survive," it brings a lifetime of sorrowful memories. Deaths due to guns leave a lasting legacy that cannot simply be overlooked in how we respond to these deaths!

Cemeteries: Killing Them Twice?

We must never take a simplistic view of cemeteries and the role that they can occupy in society. They "are complex and fascinating places that can have a myriad of meaning and uses" (Rae, 2021, p. 221). Cemeteries are usually associated with peace and tranquility, holding special positions in our society (Miller & Rivera, 2006, p. 348): "Throughout time, cemeteries have served as hallowed ground, a place where the terrain of the living meets with the terrain of the dead." This section's title is purposeful, descriptive, and not meant to be sensational or provocative, although I can understand readers taking exception. This transformation of cemeteries touches everyone in the neighborhood in one form or another, and not to mention the institutions associated with them.

This section captures a range of violent acts perpetrated at a cemetery with goals beyond disrupting a victim's burial, which is serious enough! In many ways, the destroying of cemetery headstones of Black-Americans, for example, is a throwback to when they were buried without tombstones or other burial markers, essentially erasing their names, contributions, and histories (Cann, 2020). This is not unique to them in this country's history. Attempts at erasure have deep historical and cultural meaning within the Black-American community, starting with enslavement.

Now it is likely being perpetrated by those sharing similar racial and socio-economic characteristics of the deceased, or what is sometimes referred to as "Black on Black" violence, a term that first gained saliency in the 1980s (Palley & Robinson, 1988), and considered a "blame the victim" viewpoint. This violence is not being perpetrated from outside of the community, although guns do emanate from outside. Rather, it is facilitated or enhanced by residents with the help of external sources supplying the deadly weapons used in these crimes. This is a major problem in states with strict gun regulations bordering states with lax regulations, as in the case of Chicago and Illinois (strict) bordering Indiana (lax), calling for a national policy (Wolf, 2022).

This attempt at erasure, unfortunately, is evident in a series of actions touched upon in this section and throughout this book, although these actions are invariably perpetrated by other residents wishing to continue retribution toward the families of these victims. Mind you, the expenses of replacing a damaged headstone for a family struggling financially further inflicts economic harm on them, including the time, effort, and psychic pain it brings. The economic and emotional toll it takes is further justification for this type of act, engendering feelings that the dead cannot remain at peace! The same can be said for their loved ones.

Family and loved ones may have to contend with graveyards of murdered members being desecrated by those wishing to inflict further emotional suffering, including encountering physical dangers in the process should they interrupt such an act in process. These acts send a message to these families and the broader community of what awaits those who disrespect or betray them and do not have to involve guns to cause pain and suffering. These "incidents" serve multiple instrumental and expressive goals with the primary one of seeking to instill fear and respect.

I have even encountered instances where graves were set afire requiring a fire department to be dispatched, possibly putting fire personnel at risk for harm when attempting to carry out their duties, including engendering fears of possibly being shot. There have also been instances where the graveyard stone of a gun victim being stolen as retribution for a slain gang member and their family (Cotter, 2022). The prospect of hiring security details for specific graves introduces yet another dimension to the death care sector, increasing costs and the potential of harm being perpetrated on those entrusted with this safeguarding responsibility. Cemeteries, too, have hired off-duty police officers for protection during burial ceremonies.

Security cameras are a growing business, not surprisingly. The next step entails possibly arming cemetery guards. This is not surprising since we are arming teachers (Arambula, 2023)! Arming church personnel is a step in between sharing similarity with houses of worship and installation of real-time security camera surveillance. These increased costs will be passed on to consumers, making burials more expensive. Also, security cameras and having members as part of the team can be armed to prevent further gun violence once it starts, but it cannot prevent a shooting from initialing transpiring!

Two east coast illustrations (Boston and Jacksonville), later in this book, introduce "incidents" of further violence on those already dead, with both involving cemeteries. These acts of violence (no guns were fired) have two audiences— family and loved ones and the general public to further establish or solidify gang reputations. Dying is no way out and insufficient retribution because of how a victim's family can be expected to continue suffering, defying the saying "ever lasting peace"!

Cemeteries and Children

All burials are not similar, allowing a variety of circumstances and approaches to reflect the socio-cultural backgrounds of those being buried and the magnitude of the act. However, all burials due to gun violence are upsetting and draw on past experiences and the current painful situation, and not to mention what can happen in the future. Child victims, nevertheless, bring additional significant pains for loved ones, which is certainly understandable, and strike even greater fear among the general public. They also bring an added sadness and stress level for those burying them, which many of us rarely think about and that must change to move the gun violence field forward (Antony, 2023):

> It was a late Friday afternoon when a team of men approached a tiny pink casket. One wiped his brow. Another stepped away to smoke a cigarette. Then, with calloused hands, they gently lowered the child's body into the ground. Earlier that day, the groundskeepers at Sunset Gardens of Memory had dug the small grave up on a hill in a special section of this cemetery in a southern Illinois community across the river from St. Louis. It was for a 3-year-old girl killed by a stray bullet. 'It can be stressful sometimes,' Jasper Belt, 26, said. 'We have to use little shovels.'

Burying children is unlike any action groundskeepers can take and is never routine. The experience, too, is different from a "typical burial" and can cause severe distress. When these burials are interrupted by gun violence, this compounds their experience and groundskeepers can expect to live with this experience for a lifetime if they survive these shootings. Child burials also alter cemetery landscapes in obvious ways when special sections are set aside for them, as discussed earlier, and are decorated to reflect the special status of the victims. These sections will be discussed again in this book due to their significance to families and communities and how they put an additional onus on cemetery workers.

Death Rituals Are for the Living!

Last rites provide attendees an opportunity to forgive the perpetrator of the violence that led to a funeral, introducing an overlooked perspective that can be lost in a rush to view these shootings as revenge focused (Hogue, 2024):

> At the same time, our faith traditions hold out the hope as well as the need for forgiveness. Some victims say, at some point, they found that they needed to forgive to relieve themselves of the burden of prolonged anger. It seems that society promotes an imperative to forgive. The rush to forgiveness evidenced in some very public settings in the wake of disaster can be a damaging move in itself. Pastoral disaster responders Laurie Kraus, David Holyan, and Bruce Wismer warn against early instructions, or even demands, for forgiveness. 'For most of us, forgiveness is not so much an act of will shaped by intention and practice, as it is a process, rooted in relationship, that in time brings reconciliation and peace. An exhortation for forgiveness, when imposed too quickly by well-intentioned faith leaders, short-circuits the work of lament and impedes the psychological work of grieving.' (p. 84)

What happens when an act of forgiveness is interrupted, if not permanently erased, and violence occurs at a last rites ceremony? Thus, an opportunity lost brings negative ramifications that can last for years, if not a lifetime, and may even lead to retribution, continuing the deadly cycle of violence.

This section ends on how a funeral gets grounded within the socio-cultural context of New Orleans. The New Orleans' funeral for a son killed by random gun violence, although out of the ordinary for funerals in other parts of the country, captures the importance of a "proper send-off" (Mulder, 2020, p. 221):

> While his son's untimely and violent death continued to hurt deeply, Derek spoke of Salim's funeral with a sense of pride. 'We had the horse and carriage. He had a turnout of maybe five hundred people at the funeral. Never seen anything like it.' The cemetery had even allowed the crowd of mourners to hold a jazz funeral on the premises. 'We rolled in, went around the whole cemetery second lining [parading and dancing]! We threw down!' His son received the elaborate funeral that he deserved, and importantly, perhaps surprisingly, it was paid for in part through an insurance policy on Salim's life. 'We paid $15,000 to get it done. It mostly came out of the insurance that he had. We had an additional $5000 that we had to make sure that everybody was good [that all the bills were paid].'

A "proper" sendoff is best understood within a geo-socio-cultural context. I cannot picture this type of funeral where I grew up or where I now live. Extra resources and planning entered into this final rite service. Imagine the ramifications if there had been a shooting at the ceremony and the damage it would have done?

The Importance of Wakes

Wakes are a good follow-up to the previous section because they capture the richness of traditions. Rev. Susan Johnson's (Invisible Institute, 2014) definition of a wake illustrates the importance of this event when it goes well and when it goes dramatically wrong: "A vigil is a period of wakefulness when one would ordinarily be asleep. We have gathered here today to help one another—and our society—to wake up. To wake up to levels of violence that are intolerable yet are tolerated. To wake up to the ways violence and fear poison our relations, corrupt our institutions, and diminish our lives. To wake up to the truth that the carnage on our streets is not a local phenomenon but a product of the larger society—of unjust social and economic patterns in which we are all implicated to the extent we do not actively resist them."

Green (2018) reports on gun shootings at wakes and vigils: "You shouldn't have to have security at a wake ... But in the days after a shooting when police are still in the early stages of their investigation and families are carrying out the sorrow-filled task of honoring a life cut short by bullets, it's not uncommon for wakes or vigils to become targets. Wake and vigil shootings have happened in *Chicago, Illinois, Milwaukee, Wisconsin* and *Dade City* near Tampa. And in the past 1 years, five people were killed and at least seven injured at wake or vigil shootings in Miami-Dade County."

We may question the judgment of a grieving family holding a wake for a murdered gang member, for example, if violence occurring there is a strong possibility. Isn't that reckless or irresponsible? After all, gang membership can preclude religiosity as manifested through church membership, making gun violence in houses of worship easier to conduct. However, Lauger and Rivera (2024), in a unique research on the intersection of religiosity, gang membership, and violence, resulting in an important overlap. A gang member's final religious ceremony can be a final wish and not just a request by a family, introducing gun violence at a final rites ceremony by honoring their final wishes even at great peril for attendees. Honoring a last wish is not easily ignored for a grieving family.

One attendee at a last rites ceremony I spoke with noted that it was adding insult to injury for families in taking away their final "precious moments and memories." This stance signals significant resistance to new ways to carry out last rites, which may be essential to maintain safety from escalation of gun violence at funeral homes, cemeteries, and houses of worship.

Deaths breakup long-held social relationships. When this happens due to gun violence, it does so in a matter of seconds, ascending in importance because of the circumstances of life being take before its time (Wagoner & de Luna, 2021, p. 197): "Death ruptures the social bonds that hold society together by tearing away its members. Various rituals must be performed and material artifacts constructed to re-integrate the deceased and bereaved into the social order." In the case of "good violence," added dimensions to the final rites are often called for, leading to use of death objects to memorialize victims.

Wisdom of Children Attending Last Rites Ceremonies?

It is important to raise the question that many readers may have. Is it wise to have children attend funerals where there is a high likelihood of violence occurring? Weeks (2020) notes that traditionally there have been no or few limitations pertaining to children or other family members attending funeral ceremonies, with the deceased relationship with them instrumental in shaping whether-or-not attendance is warranted or desired. Where a father is killed and left surviving children, it is arduous to keep them away from such a send-off, for example. Weighing tradition and respect versus becoming a victim cannot be taken lightly, particularly when involving children who escaped direct violence but now witness it.

Philadelphia has witnessed its share of gun fatalities and confronted its consequences on daily life (Moselle, 2021): “Emotionally, physically, the time, effort dealing with the families, their emotions, as they unpack their anger issues, the regrets, the guilt. And they all come, and they put it in my lap. I don’t necessarily get blamed for it, but sometimes I’m the punching bag because I’m the one that they can lash out upon because I’m sitting there. I’m an easy target ... Some want revenge. Some want to make a point. Some want to scare the family. There’s so many different reasons as to why these things happen.” The “City of Brotherly Love” is anything but that! It is a great promotional slogan for some segments of the city, however.

A Change of Scenery for Final Rights?

There is value in a “change in scenery” in addressing life’s trials and tribulations. This saying is applicable to final gun rites ceremonies, or does it? Why don’t families of gun violence victims hold these ceremonies away from the neighborhoods that witnessed their murder? The hope being that a change in scenery results in a peaceful and proper send-off of their loved ones. There is no guarantee that violence will not occur at ceremonies away from the neighborhood, with this move resulting in added expenses and additional time from their schedules. It is not unusual for residents in low-income communities to hold multiple jobs, too!

Chicago is a case in point regarding this perspective. Unfortunately, that city, which is not alone, experienced three injuries inside the building when a shooting occurred at a repast held at the Salvation Army Community Center at Blue Island, almost 20 miles outside of the city (Deliso, 2024). This site can be considered neutral in a location far from the neighborhood. The quest for revenge and the sending of a message outweighed the “inconvenience” of traveling a long distance! Thus, a change of scenery is no guarantee that gun violence will not unfold!

Houses of Worship and Gun Violence: An Overview

It is arduous to imagine an institution more revered in our society than a house of worship, particularly one with an extensive neighborhood history and having served multiple generations of a family. However, that perspective is changing in a dangerous way across the nation and most notably in its cities. This results in the undermining of a key institution in a world increasingly on shaky grounds and in desperate need of stability, including serving as a moral anchor during stormy times. Membership and attendance in houses of worship are in substantive decline.

Waning participation, with resulting closings, has ascended to significant importance in society because of how houses of worship touch so many different facets of community life (Delgado, 2025). Church shootings, too, sadly, have also ascended in significance (Day, 2023):

> Other existential threats lurk as well: a growing economic crisis that exposes just how vulnerable many are to poverty, an undeniably changing climate that brings more extreme weather patterns, contentious political dynamics that divide families and disrupt social cohesion, the exposure of racial injustice which enflames conflict and, of course, a global pandemic that has ravaged through our local communities. These are threats experienced throughout society, as well as by congregations already aware of their own decline. However, the threat that has particularly galvanized faith communities and shaped their sense of identity—their *lived ecclesiologies*—is violence. (p. 84)

Although I do not have empirical data, it is my impression that houses of worship ascend in significance within highly marginalized communities where establishments owned and operated by residents are rare. These institutions help fill a vacuum and fulfill a variety of community needs, emotionally, politically, and socially. When compromised, as in the case of gun violence within their walls, their influence is subsequentially compromised. They stop being safe harbors for communities in the midst of deadly storms of misery.

Day (2023) identifies the importance of how shootings in houses of worship are raising serious concerns among those entrusted with leading and keeping these institutions safe from violence:

For faith communities, the shock of high-profile shootings in religious contexts has created an acute cognitive dissonance with lived theologies that center an all-powerful deity. Those in the Abrahamic faiths are familiar with the many promises of God's protection in the Psalms: 'The Lord will keep you from all evil; he will keep your life' (Psalm 121:7), and "Even though I walk through the valley of the shadow of death, I will fear no evil for thou art with me; thy rod and thy staff comfort me" (Psalm 23:4). How, then, should congregations understand their vulnerability in the face of danger? How might this affect how they see God, as well as themselves in the world? (pp. 85–86)

Gun threats to houses of worship require new thinking on how revered these institutions are and the need to institute safety precautions for all of those within these institutions regardless of their position. Houses of worship in high gun violence communities are no longer an island of refuge in a stormy sea; they are now part of this storm!

An early 2000 study of Southern Baptist ministers and United Methodist pastors on church vulnerability to violence found low levels of violence concerns. Nevertheless, clergy indicated that violence and anger were slowly increasing, with vandalism and stealing considered the major types of violence (Bourns & Wright, 2004). Interestingly, gun violence was not mentioned. If the same study (questions and methodology) were to be conducted today, would we see gun violence ascending in significance?

I have sought to provide a comprehensive statistical viewpoint of gun violence in houses of worship but was unsuccessful. Why? Werntz (2020) argues that "good" statistics on the prevalence of church shootings are not available due to national restrictions on collecting data on gun deaths. That is not surprising. High-profile gun violence incidents tend to capture headlines when high number of causalities transpire. Thus, a comprehensive understanding of the extent of gun violence in these institutions is limited.

A 2023 report by the A. Mark Foundation on violent attacks on houses of worship found an upswing in shootings causing great alarm in many circles. There were a total of 10 attacks in 2012. Between 2013 and 2018, the number averaged 3.5 per year prior to 2019 when it increased to 11. The numbers dropping between 2010 and 2021 was largely attributed to COVID-19 closures. However, it increased to nine in 2022, with four during the first quarter of 2023, indicating a possible ominous upswing in shootings and the need to search for ways to keep these institutions safe for congregants and religious leaders.

Houses of worship are challenged, finding themselves ill-prepared to address gun violence in their midst (Day, 2023, p. 86): "Preparing for and responding to the threat of an active shooter is not part of the theological education that forms leaders, nor is it a staple of the theological canon. Violence in the sanctuary is incomprehensible; there exists no language capable of formulating an adequate response. How then might we speak of security in God, and how might we relate this to physical safety?" Day raises an unprecedented challenge for this community institution and those they seek to serve. It is natural to view houses of worship shootings in the present day because of their increased frequency and media coverage when they occur. Nevertheless, it bears providing a brief historical review because these institutions have been prime targets in the immediate past. It would be irresponsible to signal out violence in the current day without attention to violence in the past.

Violence targeting Black churches is not new or limited to guns. One has only to go back in modern history to September 15, 1963, and the bombing of Birmingham, Alabama's 16th Street Church that resulted in four very young African-American girls killed (Addie Mae Collins: 14 years old; Cynthia Wesley: 14 years old; Carole Robertson: 14 years old; and Carol Denise McNair: 11 years old) and 20 others injured. This bombing was perpetrated by White, non-Latinos! The setting did not deter this act of violence!

Day (2023), in turn, provides an historical overview of several gun violence episodes helping us better appreciate current day shootings at houses of worship beyond, but also including urban communities of color. These are threats experienced throughout society and by congregations already aware of their own decline. Violence has galvanized faith communities, shaping their sense of identity—their *lived ecclesiologist*. Recently, high-profile shootings in faith communities have challenged, if not shattered, a sense of invulnerability (Day, 2023):

> At Mother Emanuel African Methodist Episcopal Church in Charleston, South Carolina, in 2015; First Baptist Church in Sutherland Springs, Texas, in 2017; and the Tree of Life Synagogue in Pittsburgh, Pennsylvania, in 2018—sanctuaries were violated as people of faith were murdered while they prayed. This trend stretches back in time. In 2002, there were shootings at Our Lady of Peace Catholic Church in Lynbrook, New York, and a Benedictine monastery in Conception, Missouri; in 2012, a mass shooting occurred at a

> Sikh gurdwara in Oak Creek, Wisconsin; and in 2019, two deadly attacks took place in mosques in Christchurch, New Zealand. And there were others in between. (p. 84)

Readers may be familiar with some of these shootings, which is far from an exhaustive list. This overview of church shootings is sobering and sets the stage for how gun violence has evolved over the past several decades. It helps ground shootings within communities of color and what constitutes a "fair" target, which has evolved and become deadlier, too.

A decade ago, one church shooting captured the nation's attention when nine Black-Americans were shot and killed at the Emanuel African Methodist Episcopal Church in Charleston, South Carolina, on June 17, 2015. The shooter was a White, non-Latino, 21-year-old man named Dylann Roof (Herron, 2022). This shooting (during a bible reading) did not fit the "typical profile" discussed in this book but violating the sacredness of a church certainly does, highlighted the intent of sending a socio-political message (racist) to the broader community and the nation. Urban houses of worship, too, seek to send a message!

Averting a mass shooting at a house of worship is a form of early intervention, and a significant one at that! Sadly, a few decades ago that would have been unthinkable, now it is a reality. For example, a tragedy was narrowly averted at a children's church service in Abbeville, Louisville, where children were on the verge of receiving their First Communion when a 16-year-old entered the church with a gun (Golgowski, 2024):

> Mary Magdalen Church in Abbeville was about halfway into a First Communion ceremony for approximately 60 children when the "suspiciously dressed" teenager entered the front vestibule with a handgun on his hip, the church's pastor said in a *statement* recalling the ordeal. 'The church was full, with standing room only,' Reverend Louis J. Richard said Monday of the service, which was also being livestreamed. A woman standing with her small children nearby saw the teen's firearm and denied him further entry. A man at the church then disarmed and detained the boy as police were called, Richard said... 'All those in attendance, the second graders, their parents, siblings, relatives, and guests, all experienced a traumatic moment, some much more directly than others,' Richard said.

A mass shooting of second graders is an example of the challenges houses of worship face, even when they are not holding services for a dead gang member, for instance. If this potential shooter had been successful, Abbeville, Louisville, would have made national news because of the ages and number of victims.

Church security has taken on increased practical meaning and symbolism, along with other institutions once considered "sacred" but no longer viewed as such by a "criminal element" in the community. The financial costs of increased security can be significant for houses of worship with funds better needed and allocated to other worthwhile pursuits. House of worship shootings cause such a high level of national alarm that it has resulted in the federal government allocating $400 million (extra security equipment) to implement security measures at these institutions, because of the more than doubling of shootings between 2022 and 2023 in houses of worship (Rev. Boulware, 2024).

Black-American gun deaths, for example, can be conceptualized as part of a misery pipeline alongside other prominent causes of deaths within this group and community (Jones-Eversley & Rice, 2022). No community segment has escaped this pipeline. This does not deny the pain and suffering unique to gun violence, particularly since the likelihood of this occurring disproportionately falls on youth and therefore the future of a family and community.

Gun violence's legacy leaves an unerasable mark on families, neighborhoods, and the nation, including bringing an intergenerational dimension. When these deaths occur at what is considered a "safe" or "sacred" place such as a house of worship, this act gets imbedded in the collective history of the family and community, compromising the place where it occurred and challenging us to move forward after a shooting.

Church shootings have a special place within a constellation of gun violence and the nation. Shootings can involve religious leaders as targets rather than collateral damage; this act further accentuates the seriousness of the message that a shooter attempts to transmit to the outside world concerning this sacred site, which, incidentally, occurred over a decade ago (Evans, 2022):

> Is it true that religion, or the church is to be a 'safe haven' for individuals, a place where they can go and experience freedom and peace? Not for this Louisiana congregation on September 29th, 2013, as Pastor Ronald J. Harris, Sr. of Tabernacle of Praise Worship Center was shot and killed in the middle of a worship service. This situation is disturbing not.
>
> only because it is yet another case of gun violence, but because this is a horribly 'bad' death, and social and moral lines have been crossed yet again. These questions that comes to mind is: is anywhere safe? Shouldn't the church be exempt from these heartless killings?

Unfortunately, the answer to this question shouldn't be exempt from heartless killings and is a resounding yes! In urban communities of color, it is even more devastating to a community's social-moral fabric. This makes religious institutions assuming an instrumental role in gun initiatives that much more essential, although bringing increased threats.

Houses of worship occupy a unique position in our society as they address a multitude of spiritual and earthly needs that cannot easily be replaced by another institution in the marketplace, so to speak. Their unique position necessitates a corresponding "unique" response when violence enters their house. Further, those integral to the function of this institution occupy a special place within the communities. The threat of violence in "*The House of the Lord*" is too important to disregard. Fortunately, we will increasingly find religious leaders ascending to activist positions to help communities surmount the pain of gun violence, but also sadly as possible victims, too.

Social Death as a Goal of Violent Acts

Explaining why would anyone want to perpetrate harm at a last rite ceremony is challenging, with answers complex and emotionally laden. Isn't death sufficient? The answer to this question requires a multifaceted response, but still taking into account unique aspects behind this violence. The dead, after all, are dead and will technically not feel anything. Thus, there must be a broader audience for an act of violence for it to have the maximum impact it seeks to achieve.

The concept of "social death" may be new to many readers raising an important perspective to comprehend, and more so among readers with a view of death "as the final stage." This term's origin is traced back to Orlando Paterson's book "*Slavery and Social Death* (1985). Originally, this phrase referred to the status assigned to the enslaved and not accepted as "fully" human beings and their disposable status during this period in U.S. histories. Social death has since expanded in usage conceptualizing death from a multidimensional perspective.

Although social death is race neutral, it has particular relevance for Black-Americans (Thomas et al., 2024, p. 1): "Black death within the United States bears a peculiar sociocultural and political distinction. The loss of Black life, especially when taken tragically, has become normalized, reified, and familiar within our social milieu." Yes, we understand the concept of death when someone is no longer physically among us, regardless of cause. Death is much more than a biological state. When this form of death is insufficient, we may engage in another form of causing death, such as social death.

"Social death" seeks to erase a memory of someone's existence. Destroying a burial place falls within this realm by denying that a victim has an identified place and space on this earth. Eastern and Central Europe, for example, have disturbing histories of desecrating graveyards, often seeking to erase the humanity of those buried, with this action classified as an act of war (Burnside, 2018).

Tombstones are a physical artefact marking a person's life and incorporate the uniqueness of the deceased; they often have more information on them than a name, date of birth, and death. They may also contain information that personalizes the burials, including photographs and even items that were very meaningful to them. A headstone is much more than a concrete slab with information on them. They ascend to a physical embodiment of a deceased person, helping to explain how personalized and elaborate they have become, particularly among people of color.

The cruelty of destroying a headstone is the central goal for this action, with a dead victim not being the only or "primary" victim by attempting to erase their memory. Their loved ones, too, are often the intended targets. The distress level is immense for attendees at a cemetery expecting a moment of peace with a deceased loved one. It also sends a distressing message to those who are alive as to what can await them, too, if they defy the perpetrators of this violence. More research and scholarship are warranted in applying this concept to gun violence to the urban arena, particularly from a trauma standpoint.

We cannot understand violence during last rites ceremonies without a multifaceted picture of the primary and secondary goals of violence perpetrators. These acts are highly public indicators of a community on the verge of a violence epidemic or a community in full war! As in war, there are no safe zones, including funeral parlors, cemeteries, and houses of worship, all of which have historically been considered sacred sites; the same can be said about who are the causalities.

A search of the international literature found an extra-example of a government officially engaging in this act of social death. El Salvador has a long history of having a "gang problem." El Salvador's national government undertook a campaign to erase information on dead gang members in an effort to prevent further violence at cemeteries (Aleman, 2022):

> El Salvador's government took its efforts against the country's powerful street gangs to another level by sending inmates into cemeteries to destroy the tombs of gang members at a time of year when families typically visit their loved ones' graves. Armed with sledgehammers and pry bars, inmates broke up tombs marked with 'MS,' of the Mara Salvat Rucha gang, in a San Salvador suburb Tuesday. Santa Tecla Mayor Henry Flores said the crews had destroyed nearly 80 tombstones in the municipal cemetery and erased gang-related graffiti. 'Our plan is that there is no graffiti so the people feel safe,' Flores said.

Destroying gravestones is not a new form of genocidal terror with countless references to this act being perpetrated during wars (Kirker, 2023). However, perpetrating this act during peacetime and by rival gangs, and using prisoners, for example, introduces a new, although no less painful, dimension to this violence. Continued violence by "winners" signals a significant public health problem where this act is a form vengeance and provokes retaliatory violence.

Selfies and Graves

What is wrong with a selfie? It seems like everyone engages in this form of photography. Violence, it bears noting, comes in many different forms. Gun violence without question is violence at its most physical, visual, and visceral manifestation. The term "cyberbanging" has gained greater currency on the gang scene as a method for inflicting pain. This method has been around for over 15 years (Morselli & Děcary-Hétu, 2010). Its evolution has taken this method into new arenas, including the death care sector. A selfie at a grave of victim shot and killed, too, is a form of violence, although nothing on the grave has to be physically disturbed. Posting this selfie as a form of trophy brings an added dimension to this violence, accentuating hate and disrespect toward someone buried, including their loved ones.

Destroying gravestones is also a highly public form of violence. However, if we cast a wider net as to what constitutes "an act of violence," taking selfies at gravesites to mock the deceased will surely be classified as one. Interestingly, a scholarly literature review did not uncover one article on this topic. Readers interested in pursuing this line of scholarship have an open door ready for contributions! Its saliency is obvious, particularly as to why it can incite retribution that end up with lives lost.

Cemeteries as a Backdrop for Music Videos and Gun Violence

Backdrops are consequential otherwise why would they be highlighted in selfies and music videos, for example? They provide an important context or grounding for a central message to standout. The emergence of backdrops within the gun violence field is a new terrain. The terrain for fostering gun violence has expanded beyond conventional views, making fighting gun violence that much more arduous. Cemeteries are integral to historical periods and all societies. Not surprisingly, they have served as prominent backdrops for many horror films. Social media can serve a propaganda purpose, seeking an audience that can often go beyond the immediate neighborhood and circumstances. As often the case with urban gangs, social media is a medium that enhances reputations or casts insults when viewed from a local standpoint.

There is a school of thought that cemeteries must evolve along with the cities where they are based (Jang, 2021): "Contemporary cities are repeated reconciliations between past and present. Although collaging across time may be the fundamental practice of urban architectural design, one component of urban life seems exempt from the rule: cemeteries. We tend to believe, tacitly at least, that cemeteries are permanent and immutable. Cities change, but their cemeteries don't. This assumption leads to inevitable clashes in places of rapid urbanization, where cemeteries can become detached from everyday life, occupying space that could be more useful for the living."

Cities are dynamic, particularly when growing in population and expanding territorially, and will have cemeteries that have historically been on the outskirts finding their way into the middle of neighborhoods. When this occurs and the community is composed of low resourced groups and in the midst of gun violence, it is not surprising to view these neighborhood settings as fair game for the perpetration of violence, including casting as a background for music videos and sites for retaliation.

Filming a music video can unfold in a generic sense with a cemetery as a staging arena with the expressed intent of entertaining an audience; it can also unfold in the filming of a music video with an intended target and meant to humiliate the individual buried there but also their family and "crew," in the case of gangs. The video becomes a psychological weapon of terror that can also result in gun violence.

Conclusion

Readers are on their way to developing a better comprehension of gun violence during last rites ceremonies, in addition to creating interventions bringing the death care sector and human services closer together. This chapter expanded on the challenges of those entrusted with safeguarding the remains of the dead and protecting those paying tribute to their memory, including the challenges they face when gun violence was the cause of the death.

The following chapter discusses final rites and their importance for attendees. Although the focus is on those physically present, ramifications go beyond attendees to include their communities. Readers are well positioned to read a very sad, but important, chapter on collaborative ventures across professions with communities playing a central and orchestrating role!

References

Abba-Aji, M., Koya, S. F., Abdalla, S. M., Ettman, C. K., Cohen, G. H., & Galea, S. (2024). The mental health consequences of interpersonal gun violence: A systematic review. *SSM-Mental Health*, 100302.

Adashi, E. Y., & Cohen, I. G. (2022). Mounting violence in health care: Is it time to harden the sanctuary? *The American Journal of Medicine, 135*(12), 1391–1392.

Adu, A. A., Bunga, B. N., Liem, A., & Kiling, I. Y. (2023). Death, funeral rituals, and stigma: Perspectives from mortuary workers and bereaved families. *Pastoral Psychology, 72*(2), 305–316.

Aleman, M. (2022, November 2). El Salvador fights gangs by destroying member tombstones. https://apnews.com/article/caribbean-nayib-bukele-el-salvador-san-gangs-b988f02246f31c0486299b2bf4ea7b97.

Andrade, E. G., Hayes, J. M., Wood, I., & Punch, L. J. (2021). Reducing the incidence and impact of gun violence through community engagement. In M. Crandall, S. Bonne, J. Bronson, & W. Kessel (Eds.), *Why we are losing the war on gun violence in the United States* (pp. 255–264). Springer.

Anthony, C. (2023, February 1). When gun violence ends young lives these men prepare the graves. NPR. https://www.npr.org/2023/02/01/1153150959/when-gun-violence-ends-young-lives-these-men-prepare-the-graves.

Antony, C. (2023, January 30). When gun violence ends young lives these men prepare the graves. KFF Health News. https://kffhealthnews.org/news/article/when-gun-violence-ends-young-lives-these-men-prepare-the-graves/.

Arambula, H. (2023). Arming teachers: A dangerous blunder in school safety—an ecological perspective. *International Journal of Leadership in Education*, 1–12.

Aspholm, R. R. (2022). Deaths of despair: Gang violence after the crack crisis. *Critical Criminology, 30*(1), 49–69.

Assari, S., Boyce, S., Caldwell, C. H., Bazargan, M., & Mincy, R. (2020). Family income and gang presence in the neighborhood: Diminished returns of black families. *Urban Science, 4*(2), 29.

Baiden, P., Park, Y., LaBrenz, C. A., & Childress, S. (2024). Exposure to neighborhood violence and gun carrying among adolescents in the United States: Findings from a population-based study. *Journal of Interpersonal Violence*, 08862605241231616.

Barao, L., Braga, A. A., Turchan, B., & Cook, P. J. (2021). Clearing gang-and drug-involved nonfatal shootings. *Policing: An International Journal, 44*(4), 577–590.

Barboza-Salerno, G. E., & Meshelemiah, J. C. (2023). Gun violence on walkable routes to and from school: Recommendations for policy and practice. *Journal of Urban Health, 100*(6), 1102–1117.

Barrett, R. K. (2020a). Psychocultural influences on African-American attitudes towards death, dying and funeral rites. In J. Morgan (Ed.), *Personal care in an impersonal world* (pp. 213–230). Routledge.

Barrett, R. K. (2020b). Bereaved black children. In J. D. Morgan (Ed.), *Readings in thanatology* (pp. 403–419). Routledge.

Beauplan, Y. (2022). "African Americans, especially males, you know, we can grieve": Qualitative examination of emotional expressivity, bereavement behavior, and coping in response to homicide among economically disadvantaged young black men. (Dissertation, The University of North Carolina at Greensboro, NC).

Boerner, K., Gleason, H., & Jopp, D. S. (2017). Burnout after patient death: Challenges for direct care workers. *Journal of Pain and Symptom Management, 54*(3), 317–325.

Bourns, W., & Wright, W. D. (2004). A study of church vulnerability to violence: Implications for law enforcement. *Journal of Criminal Justice, 32*(2), 151–157.

Brantingham, P. J., Yuan, B., & Herz, D. (2021). Is gang violent crime more contagious than non-gang violent crime? *Journal of Quantitative Criminology, 37*, 953–977.

Bruhn, J. (2021). Competition in the black market: Estimating the causal effect of gangs in Chicago. Brown University. Bravo working paper # 2021-004.

Burke, P. J. (2024). The impact of arresting gang leaders on organized armed violence in drug markets (Doctoral dissertation, University of Illinois at Chicago).

Burnside, A. (December, 2018). Desecrated Graves: Tombstones and selfies. Urban Labs. https://urbanlabsce.eu/desecrated-graves-tombstones-and-selfies/.

Calix, A. L., & Denney-Koelsch, E. M. (2024). Rituals and beliefs about perinatal loss in Latinos living in the USA. In E. M. Denney-Koelsch (Ed.), *Perinatal bereavement rituals and practices among US cultural groups* (pp. 133–172). Springer.

Cann, C. K. (2020). Black deaths matter earning the right to live: Death and the African-American funeral home. *Religions, 11*(8), 390.

Carrico, R. (2024). *Dancing the politics of pleasure at the New Orleans second line*. University of Illinois Press.

Ceccato, V., & Westman, J. (2024). Where does firearm-related violence occur in cities? *Journal of Planning Literature*, 08854122231219918.

Chan. (2022, June 14). Morticians describe devastating toll assault style weapons inflict on bodies. NBC News. https://www.nbcnews.com/news/us-news/morticians-describe-devastating-toll-assault-style-weapons-bodies-rcna32607.

Cherry, J. (2024). Grief and coping after Sandy hook: An exploration of communal coping narratives surrounding grief communication (Doctoral dissertation, Ohio University).

Comer, B. P., & Connolly, E. J. (2020). Correlates of school gun carrying among black, hispanic, and white male adolescents: Evidence from a nationally representative sample of youth. *Preventive Medicine, 141*, 106277.

Cotter, S. (2022, April 3). Gravestone stolen in Boston as advocates fear escalation. Boston Herald. https://www.bostonherald.com/2022/04/03/gravestone-stolen-in-boston-as-advocates-fear-escalation-in-gang-dispute/.

Day, K. (2023). Guns, construction of threat, and lived ecclesiologies. *Journal of Moral Theology, 12*(2), 84–107.

De Vito, K. (2020). Seeking a secure base: Gangs as attachment figures. *Qualitative Social Work, 19*(4), 754–769.

Delgado, M. (2022). *The silent epidemic of gun injuries: Challenges and opportunities for treating and preventing gun injuries*. Oxford University Press.

Delgado, M. (2024). *Urban public spaces, events, and gun violence: Block parties, funerals, mother's day, and other community events*. Springer.

Delgado, M. (2025). *When the Lord's house closes: Church closings and urban community practice*. Oxford University Press.

Deliso, M. (2024, June 21). *3 injured after gunmen opn fire on building hosting funeral reception in Chicago suburbs*. ABC News. https://abcnews.go.com/US/blue-island-chicago-suburbs-shooting-funeral-reception/story?id=111328687.

DiBlasi, T., & Kassinove, H. (2022). An exploratory analysis of components of revenge experiences. *Journal of Aggression, Maltreatment & Trauma, 31*(7), 873–887.

Dillard, D., Henderson, H., Mangum, M., Rice, J., II, & Goldstein, A. D. (2023). Unlocking gun-violence solutions: The necessity and power of lived experience. *American Journal of Qualitative Research, 7*(4), 182–202.

Dombroski, J. (2023). About dying and death: Thanatology's place in medical curriculum. Western University Scholarship. https://ir.lib.uwo.ca/cgi/viewcontent.cgi?article=12247&context=etd.

Dong, B., & Wilson, D. B. (2024). State firearm legislation and initiation of gun carrying in the USA. Injury Prevention. https://injuryprevention.bmj.com/content/early/2024/11/22/ip-2024-045382.abstract.

Department of Health and Human Services. (2020, April 21). Managing stress among mortuary and death care workers during the COVID-19 pandemic behavioral health guidance and resources. https://files.asprtracie.hhs.gov/documents/managing-stress-among-mortuary-and-death-care-workers-04-27-2020.pdf.

Earls, A. (2023, June 7). Most U.S. pastors use armed congregants as church security. Christianity Today. https://www.christianitytoday.com/news/2023/june/guns-church-shootings-security-armed-members-lifeway-survey.html.

Evans, A. W. (2022). Guns, grief, and longing for god's grace: A pastor's perspective on guns and gun violence. *Interpretation: A journal of the Bible and Theology, 76*(3).

Evans, G. (2023). Active shooters gun down healthcare workers. *Hospital Employee Health, 42*(1), 1.

Fehl, A. G., & Mason, M. (2024). Collaborative consumption after community tragedies: Public space for communal healing. In S. J. Barnes & J. Mattsson (Eds.), *Understanding collaborative consumption* (pp. 98–110). Edward Elgar Publishing.

Fletcher, K. (2022). African American funeral directors as culture keepers: An interview with Karla Holloway. *Mortality, 27*(4), 493–499.

Foreman, S. (2024, August 27). The violent epidemic. Royale examiner. https://royalexaminer.com/the-violence-epidemic/.

Fox, J. A. (2024). Trends in US mass shootings: Facts, fears and fatalities. *Journal of Contemporary Criminal Justice, 40*(1), 65–81.

Free, J. L., & MacDonald, H. Z. (2022). "I'm numb to funerals now…": The impact of job-related trauma exposure on youth violence prevention street outreach workers. *Traumatology, 28*(2), 288.

Funeralwise. (in press). Gangs and funeral parlor rituals. https://www.funeralwise.com/funeral-customs/society-gangs/.

Gadberry, J. H. (2000). When is a funeral not a funeral? *Illness, Crisis & Loss, 8*(2), 166–180.

Garcia-Rojo, M., Talavera-Velasco, B., & Luceno-Moreno, L. (2023). Risk factors associated with urban gang membership in juveniles: A systematic review. *Crime & Delinquency*, 00111287231194717.

Gavin, P. (2023). Secondary victims of homicide and restorative justice. In C. Allsop & S. Pike (Eds.), *The Routledge international handbook of homicide investigation* (pp. 322–333). Routledge.

Gips, M. (2023, June 20). Is there a place for weapons detection systems in houses of worship? Security Infowatch. Com. https://www.securityinfowatch.com/security-executives/protective-operations-guard-services/weapons-weapons-training-equipment/article/53061954/is-there-a-place-for-weapons-detection-systems-in-houses-of-worship.

Golgowski, N. (2024, May 14). Parishioners stop armed teen from entering children's church service: Police. Huff Post. https://www.huffpost.com/entry/armed-teen-stopped-entering-louisiana-church_n_664370aee4b0f22a60f31878.

Green, N. (2018, January 23). When wakes and vigils are not safe. WUSFNEWS. https://wusfnews.wusf.usf.edu/2018-01-23/when-wakes-and-vigils-for-gun-violence-victims-arent-safe.

Gross, N. M. N. (2020). Brothers in grief: The stages of grieving for a school and its students following three shooting deaths of black teenage boys (Doctoral dissertation, University of Pennsylvania, Philadelphia, PA).

Gross, N. (2023). # LongLiveDaGuys: Online grief, solidarity, and emotional freedom for black teenage boys after the gun deaths of friends. *Journal of Contemporary Ethnography, 52*(2), 261–289.

Gross, N. (2024). *Brothers in grief: The hidden toll of gun violence on black boys and their schools*. University of Chicago Press.

Hashimi, S., Wakefield, S., & Apel, R. (2021). Sibling transmission of gang involvement. *Journal of Research in Crime and Delinquency, 58*(5), 507–544.

Herron, A. (2022, December 15). From funeral homes to churches, violence plagues spiritual grounds, too. WFYI.Org. https://www.wfyi.org/news/articles/from-funeral-homes-to-churches-violence-plagues-spiritual-grounds-too.

Hodder, J. M. (2024). "What Were You Doing To Get Shot?" exploring the perceptions and experiences of critical care trauma nurses on gun violence and caring for persons with gun violence injuries. (Thesis). University of York, Toronto, Canada.

Hogue, D. (2024). Rites for wounded communities: An epilogue to be continued. *Liturgy, 39*(2), 82–89.

Howell, J. C. (2015). The history of street gangs in the United States: Their origins and transformations. Lexington Books.

Hunter, L. D. (2024). Second-line parades: A trauma-informed response to grief. *OMEGA-Journal of Death and Dying, 89*(3), 856–872.

Ibrahim, O. M., Okuonghae, D., & Ikhile, M. N. (2024). A mathematical model of criminal gang rivalry: Understanding the dynamics and implications. *Results in Control and Optimization, 14*, 100398.

Invisible Institute. (2014). Vigil against violence. https://invisible.institute/vigil-against-violence-2014/9mmbfxetrgu4f1dc0yu9y4qaulju75.

Jang, J. (2021, December). Urban cemeteries: Evolving functions and identities. Places Journal. https://placesjournal.org/workshop-article/urban-cemeteries-evolving-functions-and-identities/.

Jones-Eversley, S. D., & Rice, J. (2022). A call for epidemiology and thanatology to address the dying, death, and grief pipeline among Blacks in the United States. *Death Studies, 46*(1), 140–147.

Kai, M. (2022, June 4). After losing children to gun violence, 'casket wraps' can help. Yahoo/News. https://www.yahoo.com/news/losing-children-gun-violence-casket-181104157.html.

Kalifa, T. (2023, May 23). After Uvalde, a cemetery anchors families of victims. New York Times. https://www.nytimes.com/interactive/2023/05/23/us/uvalde-families-cemetery.html.

Kearley, B., Wight, H., Brey, J., Fader, J. J., & Flath, N. (2024). What's in a Name? The framing of gang interventions in a city with no "Gangs". *Justice Quarterly, 41*(3), 400–423.

Kellner, D. (2022). The Uvalde, Texas school shooting massacre. *Educational Philosophy and Theory*, 1–5.

Kirker, N. (2023, May 18). Killing the dead: The logic of cemetery destruction during genocidal campaigns. *Nations and Nationalism, 29*(4), 1338–1354.

Krug, E. G., Dahlberg, L. L., et al. (2002). *Collective violence: From world report on violence and health* (pp. 213–239) See NCJ-197425. https://www.ojp.gov/ncjrs/virtual-library/abstracts/collective-violence-world-report-violenceand-health-p-213-239-2002

Lauger, T. R. (2020). Gangs, identity, and cultural performance. *Sociology Compass, 14*(4), e12772.

Langer, T. A., & Rivera, C. J. (2024). Banging while believing: The intersection of religiosity, gang membership, and violence. *Social Problems, 71*(2), 553–571.

Lee, S., & Bubolz, B. F. (2020). The gang member stands out: Stigma as a residual consequence of gang involvement. *Criminal Justice Review, 45*(1), 64–83.

Long, T. G., & Lynch, T. (2013). *The good funeral: Death, grief, and the community of care*. Westminster John Knox Press.

Magee, L. A., Semenza, D., Gharbi, S., & Wiehe, S. E. (2023). Addressing mental health needs of secondary homicide survivors through a social determinants of health framework. *Homicide Studies, 27*(4), 435–453.

Marketplace. (2024, February 12). For Uvalde families, social media is a tool to share grief and energize advocacy. https://www.marketplace.org/shows/marketplace-tech/for-uvalde-families-social-media-is-a-tool-to-share-grief-and-energize-advocacy/.

McCarroll, J. E., Fisher, J. E., Cozza, S. J., Mash, H. H., Biggs, Q. M., Flynn, B. W., & Walsh, T. (2024). Notification, viewing the body, and social and cultural considerations after traumatic death: A systematic literature review. *Disaster Medicine and Public Health Preparedness, 18*, e256.

McClanahan, J. (2020). *Posttraumatic stress among mortuary workers: Prevalence, risk, and resilience (Master's Thesis)*. Harvard University.

Miller, B. (2023, February 7). How firearm trauma impacts hospital staff. Lown Institute. https://lowninstitute.org/how-firearm-trauma-impacts-hospital-staff/#:~:text=Seeing%20so%20many%20cases%20of,of%20empathy%20yet%20is%20expected.

Miller, D. S., & Rivera, J. D. (2006). Hallowed ground, place, and culture: The cemetery and the creation of place. *Space and Culture, 9*(4), 334–350.

Montini, E. J. (2022, June 2). When gun violence overlaps funerals caused by gun violence. AZ Central. https://www.azcentral.com/story/opinion/op-ed/ej-montini/2022/06/02/when-gun-violence-overlaps-uvalde-funerals-irma-joe-garcia/7479496001/.

Moselle, A. (2021, October 14). In service and in crisis: How masjids and funeral homes are navigating Philly's gun violence emergency. WHYY. https://whyy.org/articles/in-service-and-in-crisis-how-masjids-and-funeral-homes-are-navigating-phillys-gun-violence-emergency/.

Morselli, C., & Décary-Hétu, D. (2010). Crime facilitation purposes of social networking sites: A review and analysis of the "cyberbanging" phenomenon. Sécurité publique Canada.

Mulder, N. (2020). Bad deaths, good funerals: The values of life insurance in New Orleans. *Economic Anthropology, 7*(2), 241–252.

Neu, D. (2023). Fragile assets: Street gangs and the extortion business. *Critical Perspectives on Accounting, 95*, 102506.

Neville, K., Chen, D. W., Massey, L., Cowell, T., Burbelo, G. A., Blankenbeckler, P. N., ... & Northrop Grumman Corp Columbus Ga Columbus. (2020). A cognitive skills research framework for complex operational environments (p. 0093). Technical Report 1379). Fort Belvoir, VA: US Army Research Institute for the Behavioral and Social Sciences.

Palley, H. A., & Robinson, D. A. (1988). *Black on Black crime. Society, 25*(5), 59–67.

Parsons, A., Harvey, T. D., Andrade, S. D., Horton, N., Brinkley-Rubenstein, L., Wood, G., et al. (2023). "We know what's going on in our community": A qualitative analysis identifying community assets that deter gun violence. *SSM-Qualitative Research in Health, 3*, 100258.

Philadelphia Inquirer. (2024, January 16). The stories of children killed in 2020. https://www.inquirer.com/crime/inq2/philadelphia-shootings-gun-violence-stats-children-teens-2023-20240116.html.

Pyrooz, D. C., Masters, R. K., Tostlebe, J. J., & Rogers, R. G. (2020). Exceptional mortality risk among police-identified young black male gang members. *Preventive Medicine, 141*, 106269.

Rae, R. A. (2021). Cemeteries as public urban green space: Management, funding and form. *Urban Forestry & Urban Greening, 61*, 127078.

Reny, D., Root, S., Chreiman, K., Browning, R., & Sims, C. (2020). A body of evidence: Barriers to family viewing after death by gun violence. *Journal of Surgical Research, 247*, 556–562.

Rev. Boulware, S. (2024, May 17). Church shootings force reckoning between faith and security. Observer. https://sacobserver.com/2024/05/church-shootings-force-reckoning-between-faith-and-security/.

Riley, K. (2024). Responding when sacred space is violated. *Liturgy, 39*(2), 15–22.

Roche, N., Darzins, S., & Stuckey, R. (2022). Funeral industry workers' work health and safety in Australia and Ireland. *OMEGA-Journal of Death and Dying*, 00302228221075289.

Roland, E. (2021). My father's keeper: Pathway to grief-inspired activism. In N. Sieben & S. A. Shelton (Eds.), *Humanizing grief in higher education* (pp. 150–157). Routledge.

Rosenblatt, P. C., & Wallace, B. R. (2021). *African American grief.* Routledge.

Ryan, E. (2022, July 9). A trauma surgeon details the brutal impact of shootings, even for survivors. NPR. https://www.npr.org/2022/07/09/1110544020/us-shooting-gun-violence-death-trauma-surgeon.

Sakakeeny, M. (2024). Textures of Black sound and affect: Life and death in New Orleans. *American Anthropologist, 126*(2), 295–310.

Semenza, D. C., & Kravitz-Wirtz, N. (2024). Gun violence exposure and population health inequality: A conceptual framework. Injury Prevention. https://www.cambridge.org/core/journals/disaster-medicine-and-public-health-preparedness/article/notification-viewing-the-body-and-social-and-cultural-considerations-after-traumatic-death-a-systematic-literature-review/1D9A05CBA59F14F063379B79FA2BD4E3.

Simons, S. S.. (2023). Advocacy: The hidden impacts of gun violence. Emergency Medical News. https://journals.lww.com/em-news/fulltext/2023/04000/advocacy__the_hidden_impacts_of_gun_violence.7.aspx.

Sonterblum, L. (2018). Gang involvement as a means to satisfy basic needs. *Journal of Research in Crime and Delinquency, 36*(3), 300–322.

Stanley, T. (2016, January 26). The disappearance of a distinctively Black way to mourn. The Atlantic. https://www.theatlantic.com/business/archive/2016/01/black-funeral-homes-mourning/426807/.

STAT. News. (2023, August 7). Attacks at US medical centers show why health care is one of the nation's most violent fields. STAT.News. https://www.statnews.com/2023/08/07/gun-violence-health-care/.

Swaner, R. (2022). 'We can't get no nine-to-five': New York City gang membership as a response to the structural violence of everyday life. *Critical Criminology, 30*(1), 95–111.

Szabo, L. (2023, August 31). 'All we want is revenge': How social media fuels gun violence among teens. CNN. https://www.cnn.com/2023/08/31/health/social-media-gun-violence-kff-health-news-partner/index.html.

The Guardian. (2024, July 23). Youth Alive. https://www.youthalive.org/news/the-guardian-interviews-violence-interrupter-nasir-bari-paris-davis/.

Thomas, D. J., III, Johnson, M. W., & Clark, L. (2024). You're nobody until somebody kills you: The ingredients of black death for social justice and DIE. *Race Ethnicity and Education*, 1–16.

Tributetech.com**.** (2022, December 1). 6-ways for funeral homes to connect with the community. https://www.tributetech.com/6-ways-for-funeral-homes-to-connect-with-the-community.

Tyson McCrea, K., Richards, M., Wilkins, K. V., Moore, A., Miller, K. M., Onyeka, C., et al. (2024). "We are not all gangbangers": Youth in high-poverty urban US communities of color describe their attitudes toward violence, struggles, and resilience. *Journal of Human Behavior in the Social Environment*, 1–24.

U.S. Catholics. (2024, May 5). Meet the Catholics working to end gun violence. https://uscatholic.org/articles/202405/meet-the-catholics-working-to-end-gun-violence/.

U.S. Census Bureau. (2022, December 29). Nation's urban and rural populations shift following 2020 census. Washington, DC.

Urban Institute. (2018). Reducing youth gun, gang, and group violence. Washington, DC.

Valasik, M., & Reid, S. E. (2021). Taking stock of gang violence: An overview of the literature. Handbook of interpersonal violence and abuse across the lifespan: A project of the national partnership to end interpersonal violence across the lifespan (NPEIV). (pp. 2045–2065).

Viestad, V. M., & Viestad, A. (2023). *Living with the dead: How we care for the deceased.* Reaktion Books.

Wagoner, B., & de Luna, I. B. (2021). Collective grief: Mourning rituals, politics and memorial sites. In A. Køster & E. Holte Kofod (Eds.), *Cultural, existential and phenomenological dimensions of grief experience* (pp. 197–213). Routledge.

Watts Jr, C. D. (2024). A qualitative descriptive study: What South Carolina church leaders believe about congregational active shooter preparation. (Dissertation, Liberty University, Lynchburg, VA).

Werntz, M. (2020). The sign of contradiction: Church defense and the liturgical gun. *Review & Expositor, 117*(3), 373–383.

Whaley, A. L. (2022). The cultural ecology of gun violence: Culture of honor and code of the street. *Du Bois Review: Social Science Research on Race, 19*(1), 193–203.

Wolf, Z. B. (2022, May 26). States with the most gun violence share one trait. CNN. https://www.cnn.com/2022/05/26/politics/gun-violence-data-what-matters/index.html.

Chapter 3
Last Rites and Violent Outcomes

Introduction

This chapter's title should make us pause and think of how can last rites be associated with violent outcomes, least of all gun-related? Last rites are moments of deep sorrow, coming to peace with the dearly departed, mutual support for attendees, deep reflection, solace, contemplation, and gathering in mutual support to celebrate a life once lived. Hate and fear should not be emotions that find space during these solemn moments. Solemn moments are just that! However, as this chapter bears out, this is far from what transpires at some last rites ceremonies, with gun violence increasingly finding its way into these events, dramatically shifting social norms.

There are aspects of this chapter that readers can expect to be covered; there are dimensions that will be totally unexpected, illustrating the complexity of the topic if we broaden our vision of last rites and how guns alter this ritual in high violence urban communities. Truth be told, it is quite challenging because this subject is complex, highly emotional, and awaiting new discoveries; further, it requires new research and collaborative ventures across professions, community institutions, and meaningful engagement of residents themselves.

Funerals have been conceptualized as a stage in a journey to "the other world," structuring the mourning process for survivors (Marini, 2024). Interrupting this journey, particularly when it is the result of violence, causes tremendous hardships. That is certainly the case with gun violence! Burials are difficult enough without added suspense or violence complicating this emotionally draining experience. Further, the quest to bury a loved one shot to death is not your typical experience if there ever was such a phenomenon. This end of life brings immediate, extensive, and long-term consequences, some obvious, and others unexpected. When done well, they increase the likelihood of a "therapeutic" outcome for providers of services, recipients of services, communities, and the nation, too, helping the recovery process.

© The Author(s), under exclusive license to Springer Nature Switzerland AG 2025

M. Delgado, *The Death Care Industry and Urban Gun Violence*,
https://doi.org/10.1007/978-3-031-95682-9_3

When violence ensues, the consequences extend for attendees, immediately and long-term, including loss of life during sacred rites and moments. The fallout also extends beyond the world associated with death, altering family and neighborhood dynamics and outlooks on life, such as hope for a safe life. Thus, an expansive view serves readers well in understanding and addressing this violence, helping us better be positioned to develop interventions.

Readers must not lose sight of efforts that are successful at stopping gun violence at funeral parlors, cemeteries, and houses of worship. One example that occurred during the summer of 2024 in the Susquehanna, Pennsylvania Township, where the police retrieved a discarded gun and prevented a shooting at a memorial service for a 13-year-old cheerleader shooting victim. They apprehended two male 13-year-olds at the church's parking lot as she was on the verge of being loaded onto a horse drawn carriage to take her to a final resting place (Southard, 2024). The fact that no gunshots occurred still caused a traumatic response for attendees and the community, particularly for its youth (Novak et al., 2024). This trauma, by the way, will not be captured by statistics but harm nevertheless has transpired.

Robins and Smith (2021) examine the hidden "labor" associated with providing respectful care to controversial criminals, which will likely be a notorious gang leader responsible for multiple gun victims, for example, although not limited to them. Further, how those handling their remains must ensure the sanctity of the ceremonies while maintaining safety to those entrusted with carrying out their duties. By extension, also maintaining the safety of attendees. Readers will see the challenges that communities, death care personnel, and mourners, must have emotional and physical safety, safeguarding against any form of violence.

Public Displays of Mourning as Provocation for Further Gun Violence

How and where we mourn must be understood and shape how we develop interventions, and thus worthy of uplifting. There are various ways to view acts of mourning, particularly those transpiring in public. These acts can, of course, stay private, with minimal efforts to expand who is invited to attend ceremonies. There are others who wish to have an expansive public display to allow others to join them in this act and to tell the outside world of what the deceased meant to the family, friends, and the community at large. There is "no-one-size-fits-all" form of mourning and living in highly diverse communities will bear this conclusion out. Thus, helping professions must expand our conception of this important function within families, communities, and society.

When we discuss a funeral shooting, the setting, it bears noting, can extend beyond the services transpiring within a funeral home, for example. Shootings can occur at various stages and places, such as when there is a car procession to a cemetery. Not surprisingly, there are calls to restrict who is entitled to have a funeral procession, limiting the route taken, or even limiting the number of cars allowed to make it easier for security to transpire. Further, traditional stops to where the deceased lived as part of the procession may be off-limits due to gun violence fears. In essence, what is "typical" is no longer as such.

The act of public grieving in the United States may be undergoing significant changes as argued by Delistraty (2024): "In the past century, grief has shifted from a public process to a private problem—something meant to be solved. Is there a better way?" Public grieving, nevertheless, is not unusual in urban U.S. and we can expect an increased presence in the future, as in the case of Uvalde, but certainly not limited to that type of mass shooting of children (Lee, 2023):

> Kimberly couldn't keep up with all the messages people wrote her, but she tried to respond to the ones from other parents of little kids. She got to know one mother, who also had a 4-year-old son named Zayne and had mailed Kimberly a pair of tiny Crocs with charms memorializing Amerie: an art palette, a Starbucks cup (her favorite drink was vanilla Frappuccino). Occasionally, people came up to Kimberly and other Uvalde mothers at rallies to say that their social media posts had compelled them to protest for the first time. It touched her to know that people out there cared.

Those grieving publicly often welcome others joining them, transforming private moments of anguish into public moments of support and validation, introducing the collective healing power of the group. These transformational moments bring mourners together during tragic times, including communities. However, what happens when a private solemn moment is transformed into a public one when a mass shooting occurs? Tragedy turns into support and into tragedy once again, a cruel irony during a solemn moment.

Where and how mourning transpires is localized geographically and culturally, introducing a high degree of flexibility on where, when, and how it occurs. Paraphernalia on death and burials, as per music during the ceremonial part, for example, are integral to death rituals and bears addressing to broaden this field, allowing socio-cultural factors to prevail during these ceremonies. The death of children, for example, has a transformative effect on a community as uplifted in this book.

Memorialization can be conceptualized as a key element in family and community life, helping the bereaved transition to life without the victim in the immediate and long-term. It is very important that we understand that memorialization, when successfully accomplished, not only benefits those who mourn the passing of an individual but the community as well as in the case of a dedication or the painting of a mural or planting a community garden. The contextualization of memorialization is essential in grasping its meaning and consequences. When done well or when done poorly, the outcomes can have profound meanings, while altering the environment in the process when a garden or wall mural is created.

There are aspects of mourning in urban communities that may be new to some readers. For example, the emergence of art that we wear on shirts commemorating the dead is referred to as R.I.P. (Rest in Peace) shirts, also called memorial shirts (Bordere, 2009) or "shirts of the movement." These shirts can be sold by families to defray service costs, as discussed earlier in this book, serving expressive and instrumental purposes.

Brooks (2018) discusses RIP shirts and their power in memorializing the dead, with youth most likely dead because of gun violence, although they can also symbolize death due to police violence, for example. Keeping their image in the public sphere honors their names and lives. Tattoos can also be in the public art realm although obviously at a much smaller scale than a t-shirt and other forms of memorialization. Sadly, they can also be used to identify dead bodies, which is not helpful in the case of very young children.

When these shirts are worn publicly, they can be perceived as provocative by keeping the image of the victim alive and insulting to those who committed the murder, as often found in gang shootings, for instance (Silverman, 2021, p. 16): "The process of memorializing trauma is contentious; debates over how, where, who, and when to remember are about emotions as much as they are about economics and politics." This memorialization can be therapeutic if handled well, introducing an important public symbol and worthwhile purpose. Even if handled "well," they can cause retaliatory gun violence. The fundraising dimension is compromised, requiring other efforts to generate funds for families struggling to pay burials costs.

Public visual displays of death can be conceptualized as collective mourning because of the intent to share with the public their pain (Bordere, 2009; Goodnow, 2021), which can consist of various types and be therapeutic for attendees by humanizing the deceased in a collective manner. Public visual displays of death have been generally limited to "war heroes" and other dignitaries in our nation's history. The democratization of death, if you wish to view it this way, is changed to include "ordinary" people, too.

Unfortunately, collective mourning, beyond wearing memorial shirts, as noted, can also be interpreted as an act of public provocation and a threat that can cause further violence and deaths, continuing a vicious cycle of pain and despair. Such actions threaten the power of those who perpetrated the death, much in similar fashion to urban neighborhoods that use public displays that are anti-police, which are viewed as provocative to "law and order." Defiance, if viewed as such, can introduce further resistance, undermining the existing power of those who perpetrate gun violence, gang-related or otherwise. Public displays of mourning as provocation for further gun violence are important, as attested to in this section. Urban gun violence cannot be successfully addressed if we ignore this context.

When "Things Go Wrong" at a Last Rites Ceremony

There are few events I would put at the head of a list of the importance of a well-orchestrated event, and a last rites ceremony would certainly be number one, ahead of weddings, birthdays, and graduations, for example. Of course, special days can come together. The example of a 2023 shooting at a Maryland cemetery during a burial for a 10-year-old girl victim who was shot during Mother's Day resulting in two victims, one of whom died (Shapiro, 2023), comes to mind.

Attending a last rites ceremony, whether at a funeral home, house of worship, cemetery, or a memorial mural dedication, for example, and having a violent event occur compromising the occasion and causing causalities, dramatically interrupts a grieving process. This also alters these spaces and compromises future ceremonies for fears of violence occurring and claiming other victims.

The significance of a human grieving process is well recognized across academic disciplines and helping professions (Kokou-Kpolou et al., 2020, p. 501): "Following the death of a significant person, most bereaved individuals go through a period of acute distress where the intensity of grief reactions recedes as time goes by. Evidence also suggests that some bereaves experience positive transformations of their lives following the loss." Seeing the positive in a tragic situation is important in helping professional circles and communities, too. I am not being morbid in saying this. Tragedies can create positive changes for individuals and communities, and that potential must not be trampled in a rush to focus on a tragedy.

When dramatic changes occur to a key community institution due to gun violence, as in the case of Pastor Brooks presiding at a Chicago church last rites service, showing that a positive outcome to a tragedy can emerge and be life-altering. Religious institutional involvement, as per Pastor Brooks and his rationale for involvement, is a tribute to his motivation and the sad circumstances that led to his stance on gun violence (Stand Together, 2024):

> In 2011, Pastor Corey Brooks presided over 21 gang funerals at a time when other ministers felt it was too dangerous. The funerals were all for boys and young men ... who were killed by gun violence in the Woodlawn community of South Chicago. Moments before the 21st funeral, mourners came under gunfire as they walked to the church. People dove under cars and ran into the church building. 'It was scary,' Brooks recounted in an oral history about violence in Chicago. 'I've never experienced anything like that in my life.' Somehow, nobody was hurt. Brooks decided to continue the service. 'When people are hurting, that's when we're supposed to be there the most,' he said in an interview with *Chicago Magazine* ... The funeral proceeded with police present to keep the peace. When the service was almost over, Brooks spoke with the police sergeant in the room. They invited anyone carrying an illegal weapon to turn it in on the spot, no questions asked. Complete silence followed. Finally, a young man in the back of the room stood up and pulled a 9 mm Glock out of the waistband of his pants. Across the room, another young man stood up and pulled out his gun. And then another stood up, and another. 'I decided right then, I've got to do something' ... His solution: Recruit gang members to work on the problem.

Being present or having a highly public role at a last rites ceremony, as in the case of Rev. Brooks' start of his crusade, illustrates the transformative power of a last rites ceremony, showing the power a religious leader and house of worship bring to urban gun violence. It does not have to be a religious leader, however. Nevertheless, readers can see the power this position brings, legitimizing their involvement and that of their residents, including other institutions not typically associated with gun violence prevention initiatives.

When a grieving process unfolds as expected, with cultural values in all of its visible grandeur playing a key role in setting this foundation, it increases the probability that it can lead to group bonding and validation of a life lived, so to speak; when done well, it also helps in the recovery process for attendees, which is important for them and their communities. These final rites events are arduous to begin with, expecting or experiencing gun violence further complicates this healing process.

Creating a sense of control over these sorrowful and defining events and moments can be therapeutic, instilling faith in the process. When this process is violently interrupted, and even leading to further deaths and miseries, it compromises attendee mental health and physical health. Attendees can be physically hurt trying to escape bullets and do not have to be injured because of a bullet hitting them to suffer injuries that can even be life lasting. These injuries do not even get reported by local media, per gun violence at these last rites ceremonies! Hurt comes in many different disguises. No age group in attendance escapes the psychological manifestations of such an act. However, youth suffer the longest lasting ramifications, particularly if they do not get therapeutic help, with long-term consequences detrimental to their health, family, and community.

That dire viewpoint is a reality in high gun violence environments, sad to say, and part of a community's lore. This ceremonial activity, in turn, can have a positive therapeutic outcome, bringing together loved ones and friends, allowing them to share stories of the deceased. The concept of "restorative retelling," covered in Chap. 11, for example, has emerged as a method by undertaking "reenactment through a collaborative, corrective retelling, so that in its modified form the memory remains but no longer demands reenactment and restitution" (Rynearson & Salloum, 2021, p.177). For this sharing to have maximum impact, it needs a group gathering to enhance the interactions.

Who interprets the wishes of the deceased? Odds are that there are no written instructions on how they wish to be buried and what they would like to have said about them, although I have known instances where this has been done verbally in advance. This does not mean that young people of color have not thought about their own last rites, which is profoundly sad because there is often a sense of inevitability that can permeate their life because they have witnessed so many deaths in their social network, often at the hands of others.

Their preference will be shared verbally and probably based on funerals they have attended of peers, choosing what appeals to them and how they want to be remembered. That should be unfathomable for a 14- or 15-year-old to think in this manner or to have a casket-type picked out when attending a funeral, as touched upon earlier in this book. They must dream about their future and achieving many goals rather than how they want to be remembered when murdered and buried!

Funeral Homes: A National Call for Initiatives

We are familiar with national calls for ensuring the rights of marginalized groups in this society, although this call is seriously being questioned based on current-day politics and attacks on D.E.I. initiatives. Ask anyone on the street about what is the first thing that comes to mind when the word "funeral" is mentioned. This word association will elicit a range of responses, rarely positive, with most referring to solemn and sorrow in one form or another. We may even get responses pertaining to visual images of family and loved ones coming together to provide mutual support and pay their final respects. Music, too, may emerge in responses. "Therapeutic" will be the outcome that will undoubtedly be a common takeaway, which I have difficulty putting words to. Fear and heartbreak are not an expected or welcomed outcome, and when this happens, the ramifications can be wide and stretch far into the future, too.

The death care sector covers a wide terrain with funeral homes and cemeteries playing central, and arguably the most visible, roles in most reader's mind. Hospital morgues, where victims are released from and houses of worship where shootings have transpired, too, fall within this realm. How many movies and television shows have the medical examiner portrayed in a professional manner without any show of emotions? That, unfortunately, is the typical scene.

Funeral homes, in turn, can be viewed through a variety of lenses, including as community small businesses or economic enterprises selling a service and products, and not that uncommon, pushing the most expensive ones at that. In other words, a business like many other businesses. In communities of color, they often represent a community asset at a great time of pain and need, particularly when they address an unexpected violent death as typified with gun violence. These communities expect more than a transaction of services for money, sharing much in common with a typical small business than a franchise.

Funeral personnel often live, worship, and work in the communities they serve, too, representing an element or extension of community we usually do not think about. Yet, they, too, can become silent victims of community gun violence. No segment of a community can afford to be ignored, and unfortunately, that is what has been occurring with noted exceptions. A "war" on gun violence requiring rallying of all parties, and most importantly, those with the requisite resources, which goes far beyond financial resources! It means reconceptualizing the terrain in helping us eliminate gun violence within neighborhoods and now expanding to include land for burying victims.

Uvalde cemetery activities are reminiscent of those I have seen at memorial murals, although restricted by space (Cooper & Sicora, 1994, p. 77): "Neighborhood residents often hold memorial services after the mural's completion. They may reunite there on the anniversary of the person' death or celebrate a birthday at the wall, complete with ballons and cakes. Death is answered with the joyous sounds of blaring, thumping, amplified music. Street dancing is offered in celebration of a life as much as in memory of a death."

Gun violence does not stop at the doors of institutions normally considered "sacred" or "off-limits" to this form of violence, representing a new stage in the evolution of this form of urban violence. Simply put, those institutions no longer exist! Funeral homes, for example, can experience workplace gun violence as in the case of a New York funeral home director shot dead by a former staff member (Spillane et al., 2020). The perpetrator was shot and wounded by a third party and arrested. Another example, 3 years later witnessed a Brooklyn man shot and killed, and another man injured, at a funeral home (ABCNews, 2023). Society's ills do not stop at the door of a funeral home or any other place for that matter! Further, these shootings are not all gang related, although gangs play a prominent role in this violence.

Funeral homes are often intergenerational small businesses, particularly when discussing people of color, their communities, and the few that they own and operate. Consequently, the importance of funeral services ascends in significance and worthy of support, both because of their small business significance to the community but also because of their needs and potential contributions to gun violence initiatives. For the gun violence field, it necessitates we expand our vision of what constitutes a community and a potential partner in any initiative to stop it!

Final Goodbye Challenges: Gun violence presents visible and invisible challenges that compound services at a critical time for families, other loved ones, and communities (Hemenway & Nelson, 2020). Secondary trauma, too, is ever present but generally unrecognized and therefore going unaddressed, complicating daily living and compromising a community's potential to thrive. The institutions serving urban communities, as in the death care sector, too, experience these consequences.

The death care sector has witnessed dramatic increases in gun violence, undermining its special position in high violence communities as a place for healing. The following incidents occurred in Kansas City, Missouri and Indianapolis, Indiana within a two-week period of each other, illustrating the phenomenon of gun violence at funeral homes, and how this institution is undermined in providing solace to those in desperate pain (Gutierrez, 2021):

> On July 18, a dispute among mourners at Serenity Funeral Home on East Bannister Road in Kansas City escalated into gunplay. When the shooting ended, one injured person was taken to the hospital. Two weeks later in Indianapolis, five people—including a 4-year-old girl—were shot outside a funeral home during a fight in the parking lot. The shootings were among more than a dozen at funerals and funeral-related events in the United States reported by the media from June 2020 to August 2021. The code of not interrupting the bereaved at a funeral? It's broken.

Funeral parlors have also seen their places increasingly used for extended periods for repasts because they are safer than inviting people back to homes in the neighborhood (Moselle, 2021). This response has economic consequences by increasing the expenses of running this business, which will eventually be passed on to future patrons, in addition to increasing the time period that they are vulnerable to violent acts.

Saldinger's (2023, p. 1) comment on caring for the dead summarizes the importance of this final act for society: "Caring for our dead is a final act of love: we do for them what we know can never be returned or repaid." The funeral business plays an instrumental role in carrying out this final cultural act of love. Thus, how these deaths are addressed, including the institutions playing a critical role in this final act, can be affirming and therapeutic; when interrupted by gun violence, it's mission is compromised. Again, when interrupted, this final opportunity to say our farewell gets "soiled," leaving a lasting and often unresolved negative memory. We can no longer say "what a beautiful funeral" and how we did well by them. We are also saying that we did well and should take pride in our actions to honor them.

Funerals are significant events, much in similarity to weddings. When they go well, we are left with good feelings; when they go wrong, they leave lasting bad feelings. This understanding goes a long way toward helping urban families and communities to prevent these shootings, helping the nation heal when they occur, which often requires creative responses to take into account cultural traditions. Mind you, we are not even talking about police shootings, introducing a different set of dynamics (Robinson et al., 2024; Stephens, 2020; Wilson et al., 2024), complicating the grieving process. Black-American youth are killed at nearly double the rate of White, non-Latino youth, by the police (Rafail, 2024), introducing a challenging set of racial dynamics for their families and burials.

"Hidden" service providers must be part of this help because they struggle with various forms of traumas caused by gun violence, which either go unrecognized or poorly treated (Delgado, 2019, 2021, 2025). Funeral staff fall within this group and are often unrecognized by the gun field, even when they have a formal and central role in helping families and communities pay the last respects. This neglect is far from "benign," bringing potentially long-lasting negative consequences for them and their loved ones.

Our knowledge of urban Black-American boys' grief and coping, and the same can be said about Latino boys, is extremely limited even when it is so important and touches virtually all aspects of daily life, including their education. This topic remains under-researched and under-theorized regarding peer homicides (Pabon & Basile, 2022). This can also be said about institutions central to these communities regarding death, namely, the death care sector.

The pivotal role that funeral homes play as a significant part of this sector in addressing gun violence stretches far beyond burial duties, which may be surprising to readers. These institutions are increasingly finding themselves facing retaliatory gun violence a dimension that is new, requiring careful research and analysis to create interventions with this business as a focus. After all, staff are in a business unlike any other business, but historically viewed as a valuable community institution. Understanding the range and role of final goodbyes is critical in shaping the crafting of interventions.

Helping Professions and the Death Care Sector

Helping professions that place heavy emphasis on communities can be instrumental in bridging the divide between funeral homes and cemeteries, for example, and the communities they serve in crafting interventions taking into account local circumstances. For those initiatives to achieve any level of success, they must acknowledge that this sector is part of a community. Nevertheless, this sector is experiencing threats to life and mental health and worthy of attention and specialized interventions that account for their unique position on gun violence (Sakran et al., 2023).

Any "war," and particularly one on eliminating urban gun violence, necessitates expanding the pool of "troops" on the frontlines and supporting them with the necessary supplies and backup. Such an undertaking necessitates innovative approaches to maximize potential impact. This includes "reinforcements" when called upon, covering a wide variety of competencies, to continue with a war metaphor. This support can vary in approach and intensity, taking into consideration local goals, circumstances, and funding as highlighted in this book. One size will not meet this challenge; it necessitates many different sizes to be sufficiently flexible to take into account local nuances. Further, this necessitates a long-term commitment, including ongoing support and with requisite funding to accomplish this goal.

Regardless, helping professions must be cognizant of this public health problem and assume partnerships with this and other fields of practice (Butts et al., 2015; Hawley-Bernardez et al., 2024). This approach must be responsive to local circumstances to maximize available resources and increase the chances of achieving success. This book highlights a variety of labor-intensive approaches associated with many startup initiatives. Readers with experiences in startups will attest to the excitement and frustrations this phase brings. I prefer emphasizing hope and excitement but must acknowledge the downside in order to achieve any level of success.

Altering the Scene at a Funeral Home to Save Lives

This section's heading requires us to pause and question why we must be concerned about saving lives at a funeral home? Isn't saving lives the role of hospitals and other health facilities? Yes, but we must broaden our view of local resources in helping us save lives. All funerals, unfortunately, are not alike. Yes, a surface view identifies distinct stages. Nevertheless, context, social, cultural, financial, and physical factors shape responses tailored to victim backgrounds and that of their supporters, which are often family members and friends.

This final act cannot be routinized. Human responses require careful attention to the presenting situation. Funerals must respond to the unique circumstances surrounding the role they play in death rituals to achieve the goals they set for serving families and other loved ones. This need and ability to respond in an affirming manner is essential in helping attendees to start the journey of saying goodbyes that are affirming and creating positive and lasting memories to draw upon for solace. A "good" sendoff is invaluable for families and neighborhoods, too.

There are significant socio-cultural changes that are emerging regarding funeral visitations, as noted by one East Lansing, Michigan funeral director (Petty, 2024): ""Visitation times are not as formal or stuffy or uncomfortable as they used to be. You would go to a visitation, sign the guestbook, pass by the casket awkwardly, greet the family, and be on your way. A lot of families now will have catering at the visitation. In a side room, there will be an area that the caterer has set up, and there are round tables and chairs. Anytime people get together, anytime they gather, it's usually around a table. People sit around a table, they'll talk to each other, they'll share memories. If you have just some rows of chairs set up, it's not real conducive to conversation. We'll set up a visitation room with maybe a couple rows of chairs, but then have several round tables with chairs, so people can actually sit and have a conversation. They'll stay longer and talk to the family and share their memories."

Death by guns is a classic example of how the funeral scene must be altered to take into account the nature of the death and the preparation of the corpse, and balancing the various needs of those in attendance, including their safety. Funeral homes must remain viable small businesses in neighborhoods with a paucity of these establishments, particularly when owned by well-respected community members with extended histories living there who can represent ever important glues keeping communities socially together during tumultuous times. A battle scene is not what they aspire to become because that is so bad for business and not to mention the injuries and possible deaths that follow.

More recently, funeral directors increasingly confront a gun violence challenge, often without much outside assistance and specialized training on the impact of gun damage to the human body, particularly in an age of assault weapons. They are not alone in this regard. Urban medical personnel, for example, can no longer go without formal training on gun violence and corresponding ongoing support services that they can tap during particularly stressful times without stigma. Times have changed regarding urban medicine in "dangerous" areas, which differ considerably from that practiced in "safe" areas of the country. It takes on more of a semblance of "battle medicine." Not surprisingly, the U.S. military historically had a program to take doctors for training to inner-city emergency rooms to better prepare them for front-line medicine in treating gun victims of battle (Clark, 1994).

There is a call to action to better prepare doctors for treating gun victims (Barron et al., 2022). It is widely acknowledged that doctors have generally not been adequately prepared in medical school to address the challenges of treating gunshot victims, which is unimaginable in this day and age because of the physical damage that semi-automatic weapons can cause (Meyer & Granhke, 2024). This is particularly so for doctors wishing to practice in urban areas and specializing in emergency medicine. It is not a leap of faith to include other healthcare providers in this conclusion and the supporting death care industry, too. Other healthcare professionals fall into this category, with social workers, for example, often called upon to help these families with their instrumental and expressive needs (Kaplan, 2024).

Urban funeral homes, just like their counterparts in suburbia and rural America, have generally occupied the same geographical location over an extended period of time, becoming institutional land markers, so to speak, bringing a degree of stability with them. Initially, these locations were considered accessible, safe, violence free, and essential to help the healing process. However, gun violence is now at their doorsteps, literally and figuratively. Funeral homes have had to conduct their business while maintaining a high degree of safety, an increasing challenge that historically has not been part of their experience and training (Bement, 2021):

> 'I've always got in touch with law enforcement that we can at least let them know the timeline to let them know when we are doing service' ... One place says they have not needed to have any extra security and one who says he's feeling the impact of gun violence firsthand. 'These guys don't understand the process of grieving and so the way they grieve is retaliation,' Williams said. After a shooting at a funeral luncheon in Champaign last week, funeral homes are on edge. 'My first duty is to protect our staff right. And then the second priority is to protect the families,' Williams said... 'We've needed a lot more law enforcement, unfortunately, we're stressing about that a little bit, but the main thing is protecting citizens,' Williams said. Meanwhile, other funeral homes in Champaign [Illinois] are feeling the impact from the shooting.

Williams's description of his duty to protect takes on a greater semblance of a police officer than a funeral parlor owner. Arming themselves has even been discussed, as it has in other parts of the death care sector, representing a dramatic stage of escalation and indicative of a changing world, much in similar ways to having armed guards at houses of worship. These are sacred sites and moments, lest we forget.

This "responsibility" takes a tremendous toll on them and their families, and they must do so without the support that those in the gun violence field often enjoy, minimal as it may be, calling for specialized initiatives for this sector. Funeral parlors, for example, have altered viewing hours, times of day to transport the deceased for burials, and even the routes normally taken. "Business as usual" is not possible, including obtaining police protection. Even obtaining police protection is no guarantee that it deters gun violence as evidenced with examples throughout this book. Getting a body to a non-urban location requires safety precautions because gun violence can occur in route to and from a burial.

The subject of trauma has generally focused on "ordinary" people, and there certainly is no debate about this attention. Nevertheless, death care providers, too, can be traumatized when called upon to prepare a victim for a final viewing, if possible. The devastation to a body caused by high caliber guns makes a difficult task even harder, particularly if the body is not to be cremated, which is increasing being turned to as an option (Sayer, 2022):

> 'A lot of people would think you get used to seeing something like this, but you never get used to seeing something that was caused by evil intentions and evil people,' said Brandon Haddix, the owner of Bluegrass Embalming Service and Transportation.'15 to 20 seconds of anger will end up with 24 to 48 h of hardship and work on our end,' He works to prepare bodies for funerals or cremation. Working on the bodies of people who died due to gun violence is more difficult for multiple reasons, he said. 'It takes a toll on you mentally and emotionally, we don't like to see that sort of thing,' he said.

Branon Haddix articulated the unique needs the death care industry encounters that few academics and professionals are prepared for in their schooling. Gun violence courses and workshops, which are relatively few, generally eschew content on death care provider-related trauma or have them actively recruited to participate as speakers in these educational activities.

The Uvalde, Texas, school shootings spotlighted the trauma associated with very young children being shot with high-powered assault weapons and relying on DNA to identify victims because of the extent of the damages and possibly being huddled together (Levenson, 2022). Authorities said that using DNA spared parents from having to do an identification of bodies that were severely damaged. The youthfulness of these victims made it impossible to rely on fingerprints and tattoos, for example, to help the identification process.

For many families, an open casket is not even a remote possibility because of the damage done to a body because of assault weapons. Some in the field argue that having an open-casket viewing, in a similar vein to Emmett Till (1955), with corresponding media coverage, will go a long way to showing the devastation that guns cause a human body and having this act serve as a deterrence to gun violence for others. Dying in a gun battle is not a romantic sendoff!

Recovering body parts at a shooting scene to "clean" the area, too, is an activity that leaves a lasting mark on one's memory (Moore & Kim, 2022). Those in the death care industry can consider this act as part of their "job description," an aspect of this industry the general public is unaware of because of the absence of news coverage on this "detail." Blood stains can last an extended period of time, and be a daily reminder for residents of a neighborhood shooting, particularly when a shooting occurs in a highly traversed space that is or can become a hot spot.

Blood stains on streets are usually cleaned by the local fire department. This process may differ according to locale. There are instances when a cleanup is too slow, bringing an urgency on the part of victim's loved ones to remove the blood stains, which is often done by a victim's family. Why? They may simply not want to have daylight come with neighbors having to walk on or around these stains. Blood stains are remnants of victims, lest we forget! The pain a loved one must endure undertaking this task is beyond words. Keeping of blood-soaked clothing to remember a loved one lost to gun violence is not unusual.

Philadelphia, for example, at the urging of a local organization (Anti-Violence Partnership of Philadelphia), signed a one-year $500,000 contract with a local professional cleanup company to undertake this task (Calota, 2024): "If the pilot phase goes well in Philadelphia, the city may expand it to other neighborhoods. The city might also consider working with residents to undertake more robust beautification efforts in neighborhoods with high rates of gun violence, such as removing litter and commissioning murals." Taking a tragic act, including quickly cleaning the streets of blood and beautifying the environment with community input, is an example of an attempt at community healing.

Death Care as a Community Asset

An increasing number of scholars have uplifted the importance of identifying and tapping community assets in the development of gun prevention and intervention projects (Parsons et al., 2023; Schober et al., 2024; Tong et al., 2023). Tapping indigenous community assets (Delgado, 2000) is critical in mobilizing communities to address gun violence, which is a stance that I have historically taken with other urban community challenges. These assets cannot be narrowly conceptualized because no two communities are similar in composition, history, and gun violence circumstances. The saying "think globally, act locally" comes to mind regarding community assets. These assets can be supported and enhanced through purposeful interventions responding to unique needs and positions.

The death care sector is a community asset and a potential partner for formal care providers since the consequences of this violence can extend far beyond what we typically see and expect. This partnership, as with any other collaborative endeavors, can prove challenging but worth the time, effort, and resources invested. Collaborative undertakings must embrace mutual trust, respect, common language, and agreement to increase the likelihood of success. Mind you, there never are guarantees. All one can ask is how to increase the odds of success being achievable.

Conclusion

As warned at the beginning of this chapter, there would be discoveries, and I hope I did not disappoint. I am sure that there are readers, probably many, that are ready and happy to be at a point in this book to delve deeply into more detailed case illustrations allowing application of the material covered to this point. I am sure that for some readers who have experienced gun violence in their lives found this section not to be an "easy read." That experience helps us be better practitioners and researchers in service to communities.

This, the prior chapters and the one to follow, provides a foundation for understanding the multi-faceted dimensions of the urban death care sector and gun violence. This foundation is critical not only in better understanding interventions but also in shaping how we can increase the odds that they will be successful, which can result in a difference between life and death during particularly mournful periods in a family's life. The subject of community trauma follows and builds upon the material covered in this and the preceding chapters, serving as a broad "blanket" upon which to examine the case illustrations covered in Chaps. 5, 6, 7, and 8.

References

ABCNews. (2023, February 2). Man fatally shot at entrance to funeral home in Brooklyn. https://abc7ny.com/funeral-home-shooting-man-fatally-shot-brooklyn-fatal/12761643/.

Barron, A., Hargarten, S., & Webb, T. (2022). Gun violence education in medical school: A call to action. *Teaching and Learning in Medicine, 34*(3), 295–300.

Bement, B. (2021, July 7). Funeral homes may increase safety measures after shootings. WCIA.Com. https://www.wcia.com/news/funeral-homes-may-increase-safety-measures-after-shootings/.

Bordere, T. C. (2009). "To look at death another way": Black teenage males' perspectives on second-lines and regular funerals in New Orleans. *OMEGA-Journal of Death and Dying, 58*(3), 213–232.

Brooks, R. (2018). RIP shirts or shirts of the movement: Reading the death paraphernalia of Black lives. *Biography, 41*(4), 807–830.

Butts, J. A., Roman, C. G., Bostwick, L., & Porter, J. R. (2015). Cure violence: A public health model to reduce gun violence. *Annual Review of Public Health, 36*, 39–53.

Calota, S. (2024, May 28). After gun violence, who cleans up the street? Philadelphia takes on a traumatic task. NPR. https://www.npr.org/sections/shots-health-news/2024/05/28/1245068077/after-gun-violence-who-cleans-up-the-street-philadelphia-takes-on-a-traumatic-task.

Clark, L. I. (1994). The U.S. Army is using inner-city trauma units as a training ground for its battlefield physicians. Army doctors take on medical battles in D.C. *Health Systems, 27*(1), 8–10.

Cooper, M. & Sicora, J. (1994). *RIP: Memorial Wall Art*. Henry Holt & Co.

Delgado, M. (2000). *Community social work practice in an urban context: The potential of a capacity enhancement perspective*. Oxford University Press.

Delgado, M. (2019). *Urban youth trauma: Using community interventions to overcome gun violence*. Rowman & Littlefield.

Delgado, M. (2021). *Urban gun violence: Self-help organizations as healing sites. Catalysts for change and collaborative partnerships*. Oxford University Press.

Delgado, M. (2025). *Urban gun violence does not take a holiday: Block parties, festivals, virgils/wakes and funerals*. Springer Publishers.

Delistraty, C. (2024, June 22). It's mourning in America. New Yorker. https://www.newyorker.com/culture/the-weekend-essay/its-mourning-in-america.

Goodnow, T. (2021). The silent witness project as rhetorical hybrid: Toward a theory of collective mourning. *American Behavioral Scientist, 65*(13), 1805–1819.

Gutierrez, L. (2021, September 29). Morticians beef up security as violence, fueled by revenge, escalates at funerals. Kansas City Com.News. https://www.kansascity.com/news/local/crime/article254147363.html#storylink=cpy.

Hawley-Bernardez, A., Patton, J., Meza, C., & Gibbons, G. (2024). Addressing gun violence through social work education. *Social Work Education*, 1–14.

Hemenway, D., & Nelson, E. (2020). The scope of the problem: Gun violence in the USA. *Current Trauma Reports, 6*, 29–35.

Kaplan, M. A. (2024). Working with gun violence survivors: The social worker's role in crisis intervention and prevention. In H. B. Rocha (Ed.), *Social work—perceptions for a new era*.

Kokou-Kpolou, C. K., Moukouta, C. S., Sani, L., McIntee, S. E., Cénat, J. M., Awesso, A., & Bacqué, M. F. (2020). A mixed methods approach of end-of-life care, social rites, and bereavement outcomes: A transnational perspective. *Culture, Medicine, and Psychiatry, 44*, 501–523.

Lee, J. (2023). Grieving in public. The New York Times Magazine, 38-L.

Levenson, M. (2022, May 25). Parents were asked for DNA samples to help identify victims. The New York Times.

Marini, M. G. (2024). The violence of the loss and lack of rituals. In *Non-violent communication and narrative medicine for promoting sustainable health* (pp. 35–47). Springer Nature.

Meyer, D., & Granhke, K. (2024). The epidemic of gun violence and the role of health care professionals. *Journal of Maine Medical Center, 6*(1), 4.

Moore, M. K., & Kim, J. J. (2022). Marginalization, death, and decline. In P. D. Acosta, J. M. Andronowski, J. S. Beatric, W. R. Belcher, C. E. Bird, Z. Cossland, et al. (Eds.), *The marginalized in death: A forensic anthropology of intersectional identity in the modern era* (Vol. 203). Rowman & Littlefield.

Moselle, A. (2021, October 14). In service and in crisis: How masjids and funeral homes are navigating Philly's gun violence emergency. WHYY. https://whyy.org/articles/in-service-and-in-crisis-how-masjids-and-funeral-homes-are-navigating-phillys-gun-violence-emergency/.

Novak, A., Semenza, D., Gutman, C., Heard-Garris, N., Testa, A., & Jackson, D. B. (2024). Adverse childhood experiences and trajectories of firearm exposure in childhood. *The Journal of Pediatrics, 270*, 114008.

Pabon, A. J. M., & Basile, V. (2022). It don't affect them like it affects us: Disenfranchised grief of Black boys in the wake of peer homicide. *The Urban Review*, 1–16.

Parsons, A., Harvey, T. D., Andrade, S. D., Horton, N., Brinkley-Rubenstein, L., Wood, G., et al. (2023). "We know what's going on in our community": A qualitative analysis identifying community assets that deter gun violence. *SSM-Qualitative Research in Health, 3*, 100258.

Petty, D. D. (2024, June 28). Rethinking farewells: How funerals and final resting places are changing. East Lansing, Michigan Info. https://eastlansinginfo.news/rethinking-farewells-how-funerals-and-final-resting-places-are-changing/.

Rafail, P. (2024). Community contexts predicting fatal police shootings of youth, 2014–2018. Youth & Society. In Press.

Robins, D., & Smith, R. (2021). Hidden labour in funeral directing: Providing care to 'difficult' dead bodies. *Mortality, 26*(1), 100–111.

Robinson, M. A., Graves, B. D., McCoy, L. A., & McIntosh, T. (2024). Black bodies on the ground II: Examining impactful policing policies and analysis of policing disparities affecting unarmed African American men (2015-2020). *Victims & Offenders, 19*(4), 553–572.

Rynearson, E. K., & Salloum, A. (2021). Restorative retelling: Revising the narrative of violent death. In R. A. Neimeyer (Ed.), *Grief and bereavement in contemporary society* (pp. 177–188). Routledge.

Sakran, J. V., Bornstein, S. S., Dicker, R., Rivara, F. P., Campbell, B. T., Cunningham, R. M., et al. (2023). Proceedings from the second medical summit on firearm injury prevention, 2022: Creating a sustainable healthcare coalition to advance a multidisciplinary public health approach. *Journal of the American College of Surgeons, 236*(6), 1242–1260.

Saldinger, Z. R. (2023). (Grave dispositions: Implementing alternative methods of burial in The United States of America. (Dissertation, University of Chicago, Chicago, IL).

Sayer, R. (2022, May 8). Kentucky gun violence increase has emotional toll on funeral home employees, deathcare profession. Lex18. https://www.lex18.com/news/covering-kentucky/gun-violence-increase-has-emotional-toll-on-funeral-home-employees-deathcare-profession.

Schober, D. J., Wolf, A., Castro, M. C., Slezak, J., Hastings, P., & Latiker, D. (2024). An academic-community partnership to address gun violence in the Roseland neighborhood of Chicago. *Family & Community Health, 47*(2), 141–150.

Shapiro, E. (2023, June 6). 2 shot at Maryland cemetery during burial of 10-year-old gun violence victim. ABCNews.Go.Com. https://abcnews.go.com/US/fatal-shooting-reported-broad-daylight-washington-national-cemetery/story?id=99878791.

Silverman, R. E. (2021). Memorializing pulse: The vernacular as living memory. *Departures in Critical Qualitative Research, 10*(2), 15–23.

Southard, A. (2024, August 23). 2 juveniles detained, gun found near funeral service for 13-year-old shooting victim. (Local 21 News.com). https://local21news.com/news/local/2-juveniles-detained-gun-found-near-funeral-service-for-13-year-old-shooting-victim-steelton-teen-progress-avenue-gun-violence-naryah-wright-memorial-zion-church-police-investigating-susquehanna-township-pa.

Spillane, M., Brum, R., & Lieberman, S. (2020, Haverstraw funeral home director shot dead, remembered as always pleasant. Lohud. https://www.lohud.com/story/news/crime/2020/02/07/shooting-tj-mcgowan-funeral-home-haverstraw/4689360002/.

Stand Together. (2024), Homicides are down 35% in this Chicago neighborhood. What's going on? https://standtogether.org/stories/criminal-justice/why-homicides-are-down-35-in-this-chicago-neighborhood.

Stephens, E. (2020). Homicide by police: Coping with traumatic death. *Journal of Autoethnography, 1*(2), 111–121.

Tong, G., Spell, V. T., Horton, N., Thornhill, T., Keene, D., Montgomery, C., et al. (2023). Trusted residents and housing assistance to decrease violence exposure in New Haven (TRUE HAVEN): A strengths-based and community-driven stepped-wedge intervention to reduce gun violence. *BMC Public Health, 23*(1), 1545.

Wilson, B. L., Wolfer, T. A., Wooten, N. R., Pitner, R., Moore, S. E., & Anders, A. D. (2024). "Am I next?": A qualitative study of Black college students' experiences of stress, trauma, and grief from exposures to police killings. *Journal of Human Behavior in the Social Environment, 34*(3), 390–422.

Chapter 4
Community Trauma

Introduction

Where to position a topic is always a challenge, and the subject of community trauma is such an example. I thought that the subject matter was too important to include in any of the previous chapters. Rather, it was deserving of its own chapter, and I hope that readers agree. This does not mean that this subject will not reappear elsewhere in this book, which it will. Readers, as a result, will be exposed to community trauma and its centrality in creating death care services.

Those in the gun violence field, which touches many segments of society, some obvious and others less so, can rightly ask, what is the future of trauma theory? Many may argue that the promise of the trauma field is still unfolding, with many new advances in treatments in the near horizon. Readers with histories of employment in critical trauma nursing, for example, can rightly argue that no amount of academic preparation can possibly prepare you for work in this arena (Hodder, 2024, p. 1): "Over the years, I have come to believe that one of the biggest differences between critical care nursing and critical care trauma nursing is the random nature of trauma. There is no preparation, the damage caused is generally unpredictable and survival uncertain."

Critical care nursing in high gun violence urban neighborhoods, for example, translates into no 2 days being similar, further challenging service providers. Trauma is best viewed as an umbrella with many different spokes, with each spoke representing a trauma type. These traumas may all emanate from a single cause, such as gun violence, but each can have a different manifestation, particularly when taking into account the age of the victims.

The following short, but vivid, reaction by Nicole Fitzpatrick (mother) to the death of her son, Jaiden Dixon, helps us better comprehend the short- and long-term ramifications of the trauma caused by his murder, making categorization of a trauma label challenging at best (Everytown for Gun Safety, 2024):

© The Author(s), under exclusive license to Springer Nature Switzerland AG 2025

M. Delgado, *The Death Care Industry and Urban Gun Violence*,
https://doi.org/10.1007/978-3-031-95682-9_4

> Don't *ever* think that gun violence can't happen to you. On November 22, 2013, my 9-year-old son Jaiden was shot and killed when he opened the front door of our home. People tell me they can't imagine what I've been through. *Imagine it.* It is worse than hell. You're forced to figure out how to get out of bed. How to pay bills. How to try to be a mom to your other kids. How to deal with anxiety attacks. How to deal with feeling incomplete. How to deal with flashbacks. **How to deal with the feeling that your child has been erased in the world**. Jaiden was beautiful. Innocent. Goofy. Kind. Funny. Inquisitive. Caring. And Jaiden deserved to live more than just 9 years. I love him, and I miss him so much.

It is generally accepted by those in the gun violence field that the emotional toll of gun violence can also be referred to as complicated or traumatic grief, as in the case of Jaiden's mother, bringing forth an inability to go on with one's life by significantly undermining health and well-being. Mother's Day will never be the same for Jaiden Dixon. The loss of a sibling, too, can be added to complicated grief, illustrating how losses are not statistics but actual relationships that have been severed forever.

Children left behind to bereave the death of a parent, in turn, are referred to as experiencing "childhood bereavement" and are at an increased risk to suffer long-term effects, which can consist of post-traumatic stress disorder, depression, anxiety, and academic and behavioral problems, to list several. Readers, I believe, can see the various windows through which to think about trauma. Traumas are not fixed entities with highly delineated boundaries and have a propensity to "spillover" into multiple domains. Community trauma helps capture this spillage by providing a wider lens through which to better capture and understand this phenomenon.

Not surprisingly, the trauma that invariably follows gun violence is complex, with various manifestations (Herford, 2023): "Traditional grief and social service models too often fail to address the complex forms of trauma caused by sudden death—and, in reality, tragedy of any magnitude. In Western culture, we seem to believe pain is contagious, and if we can silence the 'Debbie Downers,' we might avoid the difficulties of life. After all, if unimaginable tragedy has not arrived at one's door, it's tempting to believe those are 'things that happen to other people.' However challenging it is to see, the unmistakable toll of grief, tragic death, and social avoidance penetrates every sector of life."

Bailey et al. (2024) deconstruction of trauma-altered identity among Black men, for instance, uncovered three key themes with particular applicability to this chapter: (1) trapped by the trauma of systemic oppression; (2) identity altered by the trauma of systemic oppression; and (3) masculinity shifted by the trauma of systemic oppression. Gun violence exposure brings an added dimension that further undermines their ability to successfully cope during particularly challenging times.

It is tempting to define trauma in a manner that brings universal qualities. However, how death occurred, as in the case of this book on gun violence and the socio-characteristics of the victims, adds nuance to any definition and manifestations, as in the case of children, for example. Parents of murdered children are doomed to encounter a set of universal as well as unique challenges (Atwood et al., 2023, p. 413): "Parents often report the presence of intrusive repetitive images of the homicide that preoccupy them because of their vivid detailing of the child's death.

Generally, these images focused on the terror and helplessness of the victim, intruded during sleep, contained vivid recurring nightmares of the murder, and incorporated the parent trying to save the child." Guilt of not being able to protect their children is an added dimension, even though it is irrational and part of the constellation of daily emotions that are integral to their lives.

Community trauma theory, too, is quite complex and ever expansive, sharing much in common with an expanding universe and the new discoveries that it brings. Nevertheless, we cannot understand or predict the future without a foundation in the past, and as an undergraduate history major, that resonates with me. Community trauma, too, necessitates a similar umbrella, with many causes represented through spokes and often manifested over an extended period of time. As noted by Gahman (2024), the severity of gun violence is too prodigious, necessitating that we embrace a "historical-structural-intersectional focus" to craft solutions striking at the core of the forces operative in this country since its founding. This chapter only touches on several of these forces, however.

If one were to play word association with gun violence, trauma in its various physical and emotional manifestations will undoubtedly be the most popular word that emerges (Corburn et al., 2021). Gun violence has been equated to "*instant trauma,*" capturing how quickly someone's life is forever changed. Trauma can take a variety of manifestations. However, collective trauma may easily emerge out of a shooting at a sacred site and event, requiring a new way of thinking about this phenomenon, necessitating a grounding in this way of thinking about gun violence.

Gun violence can have a variety of traumatic outcomes with immediate and long-term consequences for individuals, families, and communities. Trauma, we must also not forget, changes the brain chemistry in high gun violence contexts, with cars backfiring, ambulance sirens, or other loud noises possibly causing immediate and visceral reactions (Gard et al., 2022). Yet these reactions can be considered as part of everyday life, particularly when those who surround you also share these feelings and these symptoms become part of community life.

The following traumas share commonalities but also bring unique elements and manifestations. Readers may have a preferred way of thinking about trauma. This section and chapter focuses on community trauma and its varied sources and outcomes. We can think of death as a physical injury resulting from a gunshot. This injury can also occur to our mental health, with a host of physical manifestations that will vary and not even be associated with this state of being by residents.

An understanding of a historical trauma construct (Ehlers et al., 2022; Walsh et al., 2022) brings particular relevance for marginalized people of color, helping us situate how gun violence has grown to shape the present and future of these communities, particularly its youth and young adult populations. Historical trauma is best appreciated as the sum total of cumulative experiences, highlighting its conceptual challenges as well as its rewards. There is no disputing that marginalized urban communities of color have long histories of fighting multiple forms of oppression, with an extensive body of scholarship to attest to this declarative statement.

Johnston (2024, p. 28) discusses the myth of African Americans having a propensity to eschew emotions related to death: "There is an expectation, by a large portion of Americans, that African Americans avoid acknowledgment of trauma, grief, and mourning altogether. Likewise, many African Americans except this expectation as a truism. The idea of the African Americans ability to separate ourselves from our pain was born amidst the unprecedented violence and innumerable deaths of the Transatlantic Slave trade. It has continued throughout the four centuries since the onset of the enslavement of people of African descent in America."

Johnson (2024) raises a provocative stance during a last rites ceremony for gun victims within the African-American community, arguing that we must eschew a rush to communal grief and mourning for loved ones or survivors. This calls for eschewing "a theology of expedient mourning" or "truncated bereavement," placing a spotlight on African-American preachers and the significance of their houses of worship addressing the importance of gun violence within the history of community trauma.

Although this book emphasizes community gun violence perpetrated by non-law enforcement, police-related gun violence is a reality, and it, too, causes trauma for the families of victims and their neighborhood, too (Everytown Research, 2021). A community trauma concept is easier to grasp when traced to a singular cataclysmic event causing massive deaths and injuries upending a community's outlook on life there (Hirschberger, 2018). When gun violence occurs frequently over the course of weeks, months, years, or even decades, it becomes integrated into daily life and impossible to narrow down to one cause.

Community trauma, we are only now realizing, manifests itself in invisible ways Lund et al. (2024, p. 2): "Furthermore, community trauma stunts community-level social and economic development and undermines efforts to promote health, safety and well-being, enabling a cycle of individual and collective trauma. Given these long-lasting, far-reaching, and patterned effects, communities with high rates of violence may be considered in a perpetual state of recovery from homicide." When the need for recovery becomes second nature, it becomes normalized.

Community trauma is compounded when residents must contend with internal violence perpetrated by residents on residents and by the police on residents. Mind you, I do not expect the police to initiate violence at a last rites ceremony in a direct and open process. Nevertheless, having advance notice of a potential gun incident and not acting on this information, de facto allowing this violence to transpire, brings to mind historical acts involving the police. Allowing violence to occur with advance notice of it potentially occurring and not doing anything about it forms historical trauma. A catch-22 situation emerges where community distress can predict youth gun violence, which in turn, further compounds community trauma (Harries, 2024; Tracy et al., 2019).

Community trauma's history as a construct is relatively new when compared to trauma's traditional focus on individuals, which makes it challenging but rewarding, too, for practitioners and scholars alike. It has evolved in a painfully slow, by my account, but steady process, attracting more scholars and practitioners along the way, with a clear horizon within view. This does not mean that dark clouds and even storms will not be encountered along the way to continue with a weather analogy.

A discussion of a topic with the prefix of "community" should make us pause and be suspicious of any simple definition and subsequent discussion, least of all interventions predicated on reaching communities suffering from trauma and highly marginalized by society. This warning comes from someone who has over 50 years of urban community practice experience. It would be irresponsible, if not libelous, to only touch upon the importance of community trauma in a book devoted to urban gun violence. Discussing community trauma is no exception, with the addition of gun violence trauma only complicating this discussion even more so. Saving victims is saving lives, which, in turn, also saves communities.

Addressing individual trauma while overlooking community trauma is the equivalent of building individual resiliency while ignoring community resiliency, and this is simply too narrow a perspective on community gun violence (Wang et al., 2020): "Our approach is based on addressing the community context within which gun violence persists, builds on community strengths, addresses all community members—rather than solely perpetrators or victims—and allows for rigorous and structured planning and evaluation." Individuals and communities are interconnected. Community resilience, although widely embraced but still in desperate need of further theoretical and empirical attention, is reliant upon collective visions of health and immunity (Robinson, 2024). What is good for individuals is ultimately good for communities and the nation, too. Separating individuals from their contextual reality is artificial and a form of malpractice!

We cannot view community trauma from a narrow standpoint. Collective bereavement represents an important dimension of a final rites response and a way of helping to concretize community trauma (Cooper & Scicorra, 1996): "The ongoing violence in the public sphere contributes to an overwhelming despair and necessitates a communal response to help neighborhood residents overcome their bereavement collectively." Contextual grounding of urban gun violence cannot be accomplished from a bird's-eye view of a good book on any community.

We must gather, preserve, and disseminate stories to understand and address community trauma (Everytown Research, 2021): "Community trauma is not only the sum of the hurt and suffering of individuals who have had traumatizing experiences. It is also a collective trauma experienced in communities with elevated levels of violence." Community trauma must never be relegated to a statistic. How can we ever put a number on a narrative of pain suffered because a loved one was killed by bullets?

Gun violence must be viewed and understood within a broad social structural and historical viewpoint. Viewing the trauma that bullets cause from an individualistic perspective does an injustice to the multiple causal factors that fueled its spread, leading to individual and community trauma. Babies of color are not raised with a gun in their crib! There is no future for guns settling disputes, real or perceived.

Gun trauma is best conceptualized as a series of layers, with each stage bringing unique and critical perspectives, but when combined, making a whole. To further complicate understanding community trauma, we must eschew a reductionist view and include other forms of trauma suffered by marginalized people communities. Gun violence may be the easiest to identify because of its physical manifestation. However, centuries of oppression, with racial discrimination a significant force, is often perpetrated in invisible ways and is part of community trauma.

It is easier to conceptualize community trauma if we watch villages and communities destroyed by war. The concentration of destruction during a short period of time allows us to witness its varied forms of destruction in a highly visual and visceral manner (Esterhuizen & Wessels, 2024). Urban community trauma occurs over an extended period of time, even encompassing multiple generations, resulting from a variety of events, some invisible and others highly visible. It is a phenomenon with qualities that build upon previous acts of violence, gun-related or otherwise, without any one person being a storyteller.

Guns play a central role in creating community trauma in this country. These communities, if anyone were to take the time to do so, have various chapters of trauma, in a similar fashion to a book. This book, however, would be about misery and despair engendered across generations, which can translate into giving up hope and living only for the moment because "old-age" is out of reach unless we define it as being in the 20s instead of 80 years.

Although community trauma can transpire in suburban and rural areas, any word association with this trauma will likely elicit an urban prefix with an assortment of images of burnt-out buildings, fires, substance misuse, and blood-stained streets. South Bronx, NYC, photos during the early 1970s come to mind. Community trauma is about a painful urban experience. Rural and suburban areas suffer traumatic events related to fires, floods, tornados, and train derailments causing toxic chemical spills, for example. These are events that have consequences that linger on long after television cameras leave these communities. However, with the exception of a mass shooting at a festival or church, urban trauma will not find greater saliency in any literature review.

Death by guns is one possible outcome to living in many high-violence urban communities across the country. However, there are numerous other consequences related to mental health (various forms of trauma) that are also operative in communities with high rates of this form of violence. Trauma, to make matters more conceptually arduous, can have multiple manifestations. This is a good point, however, to remind readers that grief is different from trauma. A trauma concept serves to capture a wide range of severe emotional consequences that help unite residents in their plight, which can be manifested in a range of symptoms.

It has been put forth that gun violence trauma is immeasurable. Everytown Research (2023) highlights outcomes arduous to measure but still altering victim lives in profound ways. In addition, positive growth can also occur for individuals and communities, which is often overlooked and is worthy of uplifting: "Trauma refers to the lasting adverse effects of an event or series of events. Living through this ordeal can change how one sees oneself and the world around them. The everyday emotional and physical responses from trauma include feelings of anxiety, fear, and hypervigilance. Despite this, some survivors experienced post-traumatic growth in their healing and recovery journey by seeing positive changes in their lives, such as personal growth and appreciation of life."

A post-traumatic growth stance can easily be overlooked when examining gun violence as we focus on the devastation it causes, as per this book. Survivors of gun violence wounds are a cadre of potential allies and collaborators, paid and unpaid, in carrying out community anti-gun violence initiatives (Webb et al., 2024). This book has these survivors ascending to prominent positions in any proposed intervention.

Readers wishing to obtain information on trauma will not have any difficulty finding ample and excellent material on this subject because of its importance and how it has drawn extensive attention from many helping professions. Further, they will not have any difficulty finding workshops, lectures, and conferences on this subject, attesting to its popularity. Thus, it is no mistake that this book has devoted considerable attention to trauma in its various manifestations, which, in all fairness, are extensive in low-resources communities of color. Community trauma has not benefited from this same intense scholarship, for example, but its extensive manifestations are well integrated throughout this book but still sufficiently important to warrant its own chapter.

Why hasn't community trauma benefitted from the scholarly attention it deserves? How mental health services are funded through insurance programs, private and public, has a great deal to do with a focus on individuals, largely ignoring the broader conceptualization that a community lens brings. The professional education system, too, has focused on individuals. Mental health professions, with psychology, psychiatry, and social work standing out as key drivers of their education and staffing of services. These and other professions face significant odds in having their respective professions broaden their focus on more expensive units of analysis and interventions.

Medina (2024, p. 9) draws specific attention to individual experiences: "Repeated exposure to violence through witnessed violence, co-victimization, direct and indirect victimization, and constantly hearing about violence in urban regions can lead to the development and display of symptoms associated with post-traumatic stress disorder." Individual violence exposure episodes come together with those of others to form a collective trauma experience that we can call community trauma.

The country, too, is individualistically focused versus taking a collective view, reinforcing individual-focused services. Thus, these and other forces combine to de-emphasize a community view of trauma. We must not ignore or minimize the damage that gun violence in the death sector causes. Its collective impact cannot be ignored or relegated to a secondary status if we are to have a holistic view of the ramifications of gun violence. It is possible to focus on individuals without losing sight of the broader viewpoint (Buggs et al., 2022).

This chapter is not long by conventional standards, and that is certainly out of the ordinary for me, truth be told. Its intent is not to "split hairs" or offer an extensive critique of how the concept of urban community trauma is being or not being applied, which is worthy of several books. Rather, its intent was to put a spotlight on this topic, although briefly, allowing a spotlight on its significance for gun violence in the death care sector.

What Is Meant by Community Trauma?

Readers have a wealth of material to draw upon to better understand trauma as a concept, its varied manifestations, and how best to treat it. I like the concept of community trauma, sometimes referred to as "collective trauma," because of how it takes gun violence away from a focus on the direct victims and introduces a broader framework of equal importance. This does not minimize this pain from individual or collective viewpoints since they both coexist. Rather, it provides a collective backdrop to its varied manifestations with an understanding that this trauma has a place within the constellation of individualistic-focused traumas, allowing both viewpoints to coexist with equal importance.

When an embrace of collective or community trauma is central to those working to help communities, healing is not just a one-way street. Elsaesser et al. (2024), for example, found in their study of community violence and street outreach workers that they experience their own journey towards healing by seeing their own healing (*"healing centered engagement")* from sharing their trauma (collectively) as part of their duties; communities benefit, and so do they. Collective healing is essential in addressing collective/community trauma!

The community trauma definition covered in the next section is simple and practical, facilitating implementation in the field. It illustrates the broad reach of this construct and its significance in helping shape the nature and focus of an intervention. Opara et al. (2020) article titled "'Bullets have no names': A qualitative exploration of community trauma among Black and Latinx youth" illustrates how gun violence can simply mean being at the wrong place and time with nothing to do with a possible "guilt," "deserving," or being a "gang member." The randomness of being struck by a bullet means that we can engage in behavior that minimizes being shot but not completely so because of the context in which we live and operate within.

There is a physiological side to trauma and high levels of stress, for example, illustrating its toxicity and far reach. Individuals with high levels of gun violence exposure will experience high levels of surging cortisol and adrenaline hormones, which is unhealthy for humans, and particularly for youth who are still growing. This book does not address this important dimension to high trauma levels that become part of daily living in high-violence communities because of lack of space. Readers have an abundance of material to better comprehend its physiological ramifications.

Community Trauma Definition

Clearly, this is not a book on community trauma. Nevertheless, we cannot ignore its influential presence in shaping this book. I struggled with providing a definition true to its meaning and practical enough to use in research and practice, whether it is in "regular" practice or practice in the deathcare sector. I also struggled with this task when I wrote (Delgado, 2022), "*Urban Gun Violence: Self-help organizations as healing sites, catalysts for change, and collaborative partners*." I like to rationalize that struggle is always good for the soul, so to speak. Nevertheless, it is painful while you are in the midst of this struggle for the soul to be hyperbolic!

Community trauma's reach is broad and does not lend itself to simplistic views. We must remember that isolating gun violence from other forces and acts, such as severe economic challenges and community violence, is artificial and denies the reality youth and others face in daily life. Life is never that simple! That stance does not preclude us from focusing on gun violence, but we cannot separate this form of violence from racial trauma (Armstrong & Carlson, 2019); to do so does an injustice to both. Sadly, but not surprisingly, a victim's race, more so if they were Black, is a strong predictor of less, rather than more, public support in the recovery process (Berryessa et al., 2023). Lack of support makes a difficult situation even more arduous as a result.

I, and countless others in the gun violence field, subscribe to Pinderhughes et al. (2015) definition of collective/community trauma, for good reasons. They define this trauma as "an aggregate of trauma experienced by community members or an event that impacts a few people but has structural and social traumatic consequences." This definition stresses concrete ramifications that can be identified and measured at a collective level. It does not narrowly conceptualize these consequences and lose sight of how a community is impacted. We must remember that other deleterious consequences are present when discussing marginalized communities of color, compounding gun violence outcomes.

There is a desperate call for community trauma-informed research to guide public health and health inequities (Johnson-Lawrence et al., 2024), with findings crafting potential interventions. Simply put, more research is needed! For this research to be successful in setting a foundation and its parameters, it will require broad community participation, including segments having experienced individual trauma and institutions we normally would not consider, such as the death care sector.

Trauma-informed interventions must be crafted to take into account the death care sector, as in the case of religious institutions within the Latino community (Hernandez, 2024), for example. These types of efforts, again, cannot take a cookie-cutter approach because of the unique aspects that the death sector brings. Nevertheless, the spirit and values behind these efforts can be universal, as touched upon throughout this book, with local circumstances dictating how they are operationalized. I cannot stress that enough, particularly when thinking about community trauma.

Key Elements of Community Trauma

A community trauma concept must be all-encompassing, but by doing so it becomes unwieldy and difficult to operationalize for practice. That, unfortunately, can be true in a rush to paint a broad picture of a community's sufferings. Statistics, unfortunately, often take a front and center stage in setting such a portrait. However, being able to operationalize a concept with multiple perspectives or nuances is equally important as our ability to put it into practice. In fact, the latter would not be possible without the former.

The concept of community trauma can go by many different terms, complicating the development of this construct, such as community distress, community violence, historical trauma, neighborhood trauma, intergenerational trauma, collective trauma, and vicarious community trauma, to list several of the more popular terms. The following case illustrates how boundaries between these different terms are arduous to differentiate. It is not unusual for some families, as in the case of Philadelphia, Pennsylvania's Movita Johnson-Harrrell (Dean, 2024), that they can count on losing multiple generations to gun violence (intergenerational cycle of trauma), compromising numerous holidays and key community institutions while touching upon multiple ways of categorizing her experience:

> For or most people, Easter is a time for celebration, a reflection on rebirth. For Movita Johnson-Harrell, the holiday evokes feelings that are much more somber. It was on Easter Sunday in 1975 when gun violence claimed the first of five lives in her immediate family. From that night on, violence has been a constant. Her father, her brother, a cousin, and her two sons all have been killed since that day. The losses suffered by Johnson-Harrell's family illustrate how deeply gun violence has affected Black communities in Philadelphia and in other cities throughout America across generations. It bears noting that in Philadelphia 80% of that city's homicides involved Black victims.

Researchers and practitioners, as a result, need to account for universal factors without sacrificing sufficient flexibility to consider local circumstances in a rush to attach a trauma label. Community trauma calls for a corresponding community perspective or focus, which is not a conceptual leap (Johnson-Lawrence et al., 2024; Urban Health Institute, 2015). This gun violence lens brings potential rewards as well as challenges, particularly for those of us used to thinking of trauma from an individualistic standpoint. Helping professions appreciate the varied ways individual trauma can get caused and manifested. The same cannot be said about community trauma.

The broader picture that community trauma brings, although tremendously advantageous to solving local problems, challenges us to conceptualize broader interventions, particularly ones in new arenas. This must not dissuade us from seeking innovative interventions. This introduces creative thinking of how to help communities, including innovative strategies, particularly so when we are prepared to develop strategies that take into account neighborhood history, circumstances, and characteristics, daring us to think "out of the box."

Creativity, I would contend, is not a trait or quality that is encouraged in higher education. In fact, the most creative people I know are young children. The least creative? I would venture to say it would be doctoral students who must please four individuals in their dissertation defense! I like to say that doctoral programs share much similarity to prisons, with saying the "right" thing at a parole board hearing dictating whether or not you go free!

We must not forget that the most appropriate approach to addressing community pain, as manifested through trauma, necessitates viewing healing from a community standpoint, which invariably involves "reconciliation and forgiveness, justice and truth-telling," considered the core of any form of healing, with very religious overtones, I might add, whether it is at the individual or community level. These qualities are often seen as the backbone to any healing process—be it individual or communal, nationally or internationally (Ngwenya & Ngwenya, 2018).

Public Violence and Guns

Mass shootings, as is often the case with semi-assault weapons, can cause high numbers of casualties and severe injuries, which cannot be solely measured by the number of deaths and the nature and extent of physical injuries. Verbal violence (severe cursing, insults, and threats), for instance, is rarely included within this concept, yet it is present and may have even led to public violence; it, too, can hurt. There are psychological manifestations (trauma), which can reach out beyond those at the sites of these shootings. That makes the ramifications of public violence extensive and arduous to measure, a key element in any effort to obtain research and programmatic funds, for example.

Nevertheless, we often cannot wait for authorities to make the necessary commitments before communities respond. For community outsiders, particularly ones that developed their image of this entity through local public media ("*crime beat*"), it is relatively easy to create the impression that violence is rampant with few escaping its direct physical consequences. However, the truth is closer to only a relatively small number of residents are committing these crimes, with many law-abiding but still suffering the myriad of consequences.

Community trauma is public violence and trauma combined, and most importantly, it can extend far beyond those in attendance at an event and who are directly physically injured. Causing wide "public pain" is the goal of these violent acts. This broad context is not meant to minimize the individual suffering experienced within a community, and in this case related to guns, because this is usually the way we think about this construct. Thus, community trauma does not diminish the importance of the various forms of individual trauma that exist. Rather, this concept provides practitioners and academics with a different lens and the need to undertake assorted actions to address it. Addressing community trauma is not meant to substitute for a variety of individual traumas. Rather, it seeks to complement.

It would not be extraordinary to ask anyone on the street what they think of when community trauma, guns, and adolescents are mentioned, expecting a range of reactions with most centered on emotional fragility of various kinds, with an increased sense of fears of varied kinds. When we think of community trauma in a broader manner, it opens the door for a better grasp of how gun violence can be so devastating (Duwe, 2020), undermining the basic social fabric of a neighborhood. Bruns et al. (2024), for example, studied adolescent community exposure to gun violence and educational aspirations. Adolescents exposed to gun violence had lower high school graduation expectations, which should not be surprising. To make it even more challenging, those under the age of 12 with exposure to gun violence also have a higher likelihood of carrying a gun for protection.

Equally important is that this type of exposure does not have to be witnessed or experienced firsthand to shape these aspirations, indicative of the myriad of ways that we must broaden our conceptualizations of community trauma. This is a very important observation for the field. Knowing victims from a distance, so to speak, or hearing about someone they did not know personally can shape a narrative that creates the odds against them in life (Bruns et al., 2024). Hearing stories of gun violence at a sacred event is an example of how this "news" travels everywhere and is the subject of serious discussion with other adolescents about how life can be dramatically altered by a bullet intended for them or someone else.

Conclusion

This chapter sought to aid readers in developing an appreciation of the importance of community perspectives on trauma because of how gun violence at solemn events has generally been conceptualized at an individual level. This stance does not take away from individual traumas, which are significant. The slogan "It takes a Village" comes to mind on how to proceed in addressing community trauma (Hall-Hipkins et al., 2024). It does help us grasp gun violence manifestations beyond a simplistic view of victim and perpetrator and life and death. This perspective does not take away from the more conventional views of trauma, which can consist of multiple types. A community trauma view, however, offers a foundation upon which individual traumas can rest without losing sight of the broader consequences of gun violence.

Readers have a grounding in a definition of community trauma and its broad parameters that facilitates practical application with countless scars that residents can easily understand by how it gets manifested when discussing gun violence. This mental state permeates widely, with manifestations easily overlooked by external authorities in crafting interventions. This viewpoint heightens expectations for addressing the multiple layers of this community public health problem, building upon the various forms of individually focused trauma. **Part II** that follows consists of four case illustrations of various lengths on gun violence in funeral homes, cemeteries, and houses of worship. Violence takes various forms but is still intended to perpetrate harm. These illustrations provide an opportunity to tie material from **Part I**.

References

Armstrong, M., & Carlson, J. (2019). Speaking of trauma: The race talk, the gun violence talk, and the racialization of gun trauma. *Palgrave Communications, 5*(1) .

Atwood, J. D., Schaefer-Schiumo, K., & Russo, A. (2023). The ultimate trauma: A murdered child counseling considerations. *The Family Journal, 31*(3), 406–416.

Bailey, A., Bailey, R., Newman, G., Barrett, A., Nguyen, M., & Lindsay, J. (2024). Deconstructing the trauma-altered identity of Black men. *Journal of Child & Adolescent Trauma, 17*(3), 999–1012.

Berryessa, C. M., Sierra-Arevalo, M., & Semenza, D. C. (2023). Portrayals of gun violence victimization and public support for firearm policies: An experimental analysis. *Journal of Experimental Criminology, 19*(4).

Bruns, A., Aubel, A. J., Zhang, X., Buggs, S. A., & Kravitz-Wirtz, N. (2024). Community exposure to gun homicide and adolescents' educational aspirations. *Journal of Adolescence*. in press.

Buggs, S. A., Kravitz-Wirtz, N. D., & Lund, J. J. (2022). Social and structural determinants of community firearm violence and community trauma. *The Annals of the American Academy of Political and Social Science, 704*(1), 224–241.

Cooper, M., & Sciorra, J. (1996). *R.I.P. memorial wall art*. Thames & Hudson.

Corburn, J., Boggan, D., Muttaqi, K., Vaughn, S., Houston, J., Thibodeaux, J., & Muhammad, B. (2021). A healing-centered approach to preventing urban gun violence: The advance peace model. *Humanities and Social Sciences Communications, 8*(1), 1–7.

Dean, M. M. (2024, December 5). The intergenerational fallout of gun violence. The Trace. https://www.thetrace.org/2024/12/gun-homicide-structural-racism-philly/.

Delgado, M. (2022). *Urban gun violence: Self-help organizations as healing sites, catalysts for change and collaborative partners*. Oxford University Press.

Duwe, G. (2020). Patterns and prevalence of lethal mass violence. *Criminology & Public Policy, 19*(1), 17–35.

Ehlers, C. L., Yehuda, R., Gilder, D. A., Bernert, R., & Karriker-Jaffe, K. J. (2022). Trauma, historical trauma, PTSD and suicide in an American Indian community sample. *Journal of Psychiatric Research, 156*, 214–220.

Elsaesser, C., Vasquez Reyes, M., Fairchild, E., Santiago, J., Lopez, D., & Courts, D. (2024). "Being someone who can buffer the pains of life": Street outreach worker perspectives on supporting youths' healing from community violence. *Clinical Social Work Journal*, 1–12.

Esterhuizen, E., & Wessels, W. (2024). The trauma of war: Reflecting on aspects of fear, loss, but also disempowerment of the enemy (hope) in the book of Nahum. *Pharos Journal of Theology, 105*(1).

Everytown Research. (2021, May 27). Invisible wounds: Gun violence and community trauma theory among Black Americans. https://everytownresearch.org/report/invisible-woundsgun-violence-and-community-trauma-among-black-americans/.

Everytown Support Fund. (2023, June 1). Meet the survivors who support other survivors. https://everytownsupportfund.org/meet-the-survivors-who-support-other-survivors/.

Everytown for Gun Safety. (2024, September 15). What the cost of gun violence costs us. https://www.everytown.org/what-the-cost-of-gun-violence-costs-us/.

Gahman, L. (2024). Alienation flows through the barrel of a gun: Despair, mass shootings, and suicide in an American settler colony. *Human Geography, 17*(1), 67–75.

Gard, A. M., Brooks-Gunn, J., McLanahan, S. S., Mitchell, C., Monk, C. S., & Hyde, L. W. (2022). Deadly gun violence, neighborhood collective efficacy, and adolescent neurobehavioral outcomes. *PNAS Nexus, 1*(3), pgac061.

Hall-Hipkins, C., Angalet, G., & Dillard, D. (2024). It takes a village: Moving from unaligned action to collective impact. *Delaware Journal of Public Health, 1*.

Harries. (2024). Youth gun violence. *Pediatric Annals, 53*(6), e197–e199.

Herford, K. N. (2023, January 9). Creating sanctuary for the tragically bereaved. Thirteen PBS. https://www.thirteen.org/blog-post/creating-sanctuary-bereaved/.

Hernandez, V. (2024). Bridging the gap between spirituality and mental health: The need for trauma-informed ministries within Latino communities. *Journal of Religion & Spirituality in Social Work: Social Thought, 43*(2), 169–181.

Hirschberger, G. (2018). Collective trauma and the social construction of meaning. *Frontiers in Psychology, 9*, 1441.

Hodder, J. M. (2024). *"What were you doing to get shot?" Exploring the perceptions and experiences of critical care nurses and gun violence and carung for persons with gun injuries*. Master's Thesis. York University, Toronto, Canada.

Johnson, C. D. (2024). Grave preaching: Homiletical violence in the face of grief. *Theology Today, 81*(1), 27–34.

Johnson-Lawrence, V., Sneed, R., Dotson, K., Njoroge, M., & Pugh, P. (2024). *Trauma-informed approaches and community engagement: Community engaged research (CEnR) and programming for public health and health inequities*. RTI Press.

Johnston, C. D. (2024). Grave preaching: Homiletical violence in the face of grief. *Theology Today, 81*(1), 27–34.

Lund, J. I., Aubal, A. J., & Buggs, S. A. (2024). Community-based violence intervention in the aftermass of homicide: Community violence prevention specailists' proximity to and perspectives on community safety and healing. *Homicide Studies, 29*(1).

Medina, B. (2024). "Bro, ours is going untreated, ours is going unnoticed, and it's fucked up": Community trauma and education (Master's Thesis, California State University San Marcos, CA).

Ngwenya, D., & Ngwenya, D. (2018). Community trauma healing—theory and practice. Healing the wounds of Gukurahundi in Zimbabwe: A participatory action research project. (pp. 63–94).

Opara, I., Lardier, D. T., Metzger, I., Herrera, A., Franklin, L., Garcia-Reid, P., & Reid, R. J. (2020). "Bullets have no names": A qualitative exploration of community trauma among Black and Latinx youth. *Journal of Child and Family Studies, 29*, 2117–2129.

Pinderhughes, H., Davis, R., & Williams, M. (2015). Adverse community experiences and resilience: A framework for addressing and preventing community trauma. In J. D. Osofsky & B. M. Groves (Eds.), *Violence and trauma in the lives of children: Prevention and intervention* (pp. 215–234). Praeger/ABC-CLIO.

Robinson, L. T. (2024). History matters exploring intergenerational trauma and human connection—a community engagement project. *Expressive Therapies Capstone Theses, 783*. .

Tracy, B. M., Smith, R. N., Miller, K., Clayton, E., Bailey, K., Gerrin, C., et al. (2019). Community distress predicts youth gun violence. *Journal of Pediatric Surgery, 54*(11), 2375–2381.

Urban Health Institute. (2015). Urban health. Healing together: Community-level trauma. Its causes, consequences, and solutions. Johns Hopkins University. https://urbanhealth.jhu.edu/sites/default/files/2023-05/sdh-2015-brief-1.pdf.

Walsh, M. J., Abernathy, R. P. T., & Levers, L. L. (2022). Historical trauma and trauma-affected communities. In L. López Levers (Ed.), *Trauma counseling, second edition theories and interventions for managing trauma, stress, crisis, and disaster* (2nd ed., pp. 297–310). Springer.

Wang, E. A., Riley, C., Wood, G., Greene, A., Horton, N., Williams, M., et al. (2020). Building community resilience to prevent and mitigate community impact of gun violence: Conceptual framework and intervention design. *BMJ Open, 10*(10), e040277.

Webb, P. B., Jimenez, J., Elder, A., Cotte, A. O., Ravichandran, A., Holbrook, E., et al. (2024). Exploring lived experiences of gunshot wound survivors: A key to ethnographically informed public health interventions for curbing firearm violence. *Injury, 55*(2), 111240.

Part II
Case Illustrations

Chapter 5
Chicago, Illinois (Funeral Parlor)

Introduction

Readers must not read this and the other three chapters that follow without examining their own tendencies to show emotions or reactions at last rites ceremonies. My experiences, which admittedly have been primarily of Latino and Black-American funerals, exposed me to a range of intense emotions that carried out into the community at large. When attending White, non-Latino ceremonies, there is a general absence of highly visible emotions and a greater degree of predictability as to what will follow. The contrast is quite stark and significant.

Part II places heavy emphasis on illustrations of various aspects of the death care sector, helping to concretize how key concepts are realized. Each chapter focuses on a particular segment of the death care sector city's cemeteries, funeral homes, or houses of worship. This facilitates developing a better appreciation of the death sector and how gun violence has dramatically changed the local scene at these sites. Collectively, these four chapters paint a more well-rounded portrait of the death sector: This chapter (Chicago, Illinois); Chap. 6 (Boston, Massachusetts); Chap. 7 (Pittsburgh, Pennsylvania); and finally Chap. 8 (Jacksonville, Florida).

This section attempts to facilitate the application of theory, setting a foundation for the final section's coverage of research, education, and practice. Readers are reminded that case illustrations are just that—illustrations. Unlike their case study counterparts that provide in-depth treatment of an issue with extensive coverage. Illustrations provide a snapshot view rather than a highly detailed portrait. Illustrations also allow a greater number of examples to be put forth in a limited amount of space, highlighting the devastation of these acts on mourners, their families, and communities, including those in the death care sector.

I have a deep fondness for case illustrations. As a very practical person, I want to know the "bottom line" or the "so what" of a topic. Statistics and theory bring little meaning without putting faces and stories to this information (contextual

© The Author(s), under exclusive license to Springer Nature Switzerland AG 2025
M. Delgado, *The Death Care Industry and Urban Gun Violence*, https://doi.org/10.1007/978-3-031-95682-9_5

grounding), although acknowledging the important role they can play in crafting solutions to complex problems. Chicago is best appreciated through a case illustration lens, synthesizing various forms of information to shape a collective portrait that not only informs us but also serves to energize us in the process.

During the initial conceptualization of this book, I never doubted which case illustration would start this portion of the book. This is not because I have a strong dislike for this city. On the contrary, truth be told, I am very fond of Chicago, taking its place behind New York City, my birthplace and where I spent my formative years. I graduated from the University of Illinois, Urbana, and my closest friends were almost all from Chicago and Latinos (Mexicans and Puerto Ricans). They grew up on Division Street (South Side) and attended Tooley High School, which closed in 1974.

I would visit Chicago (139 miles) every school break and stay with them. Since then, I have traveled back to Chicago on countless occasions to do consultations, workshops, and give conference speeches. I have also brought my family there on various vacations. Thus, Chicago is more than a geographical entity on a map and a backdrop to horrific gun violence acts! Needless to say, it is a city that is near and dear to me.

Sadly, Chicago can easily be the focus of this entire book on gun violence at funeral homes, cemeteries, and houses of worship. Chicago can also sadly take its place against any other city in the country, including New York, which has a considerably larger population. Thus, my "adopted hometown" receives considerable attention in this book for good reasons. There are so many different ways to think about the likelihood of premature death in Chicago, which is not a rare occasion in some of its most dangerous neighborhoods. Devaney's (2022) study titled "*Death by Abandonment: Understanding North Lawndale's Historically High Homicide Rate*" illustrates the potential of a comprehensive view of key economic forces being operative in causing this state of being, including neglect by City government.

We cannot discuss Chicago summers without attention to gun violence. I have a propensity to associate Memorial Day with the start of celebrations but also, quite sadly, the start of the shooting season (Reeping & Hemenway, 2020), and a thunderstorm of bullets to spoil that time of the year for those seeking relief from the misery of heat and humidity (Kotlowitz, 2020). Summer is a season that many of us look forward to. Unfortunately, it is also a period when gun violence increases in frequency in cities across the nation, bringing fear in high-violence communities as more residents venture out of their homes and gather in public spaces such as parks and playgrounds, for example.

One summer day in Chicago witnessed a series of shootings causing 7 deaths and 33 wounded, with the youngest death victim being a 14-year-old who was looking forward to his first day of high school, and tragically, it was not to be (Hutchinson, 2023). Chicago, three weekends earlier, also had a deadly period with 5 fatalities and 47 injured in 29 separate incidents with victims aged 20–33 years of age (Masterson, 2023). These statistics do not capture those who visually witnessed or heard these shootings, or the heartaches of those related to the victims and will need to attend funerals.

Chicago, over the 2024 July 4th weekend, had more than 100 shootings, resulting in 19 deaths. This figure occurred against a backdrop (as of June 24, 2024) of over 1105 shootings representing a 6% reduction since that date last year and a 12% reduction from 2022, to highlight a positive trend! Nevertheless, that would not be the sentiments of those killed and their loved ones who must prepare for burials and life without them, having to rely on memories and artifacts symbolizing their lives rather than having them present (CNN, 2024). Apprehension of being injured or killed by a bullet can also apply to other urban areas of the country, including Boston, Jacksonville, and Pittsburgh, as highlighted in this book, and others escaping in-depth attention, including small towns and cities. This is a tremendously sad commentary on the state of this country and its urban centers.

Why is summer such a violent season? Seewer (2024) identifies a convergence of factors, such as school vacations, more social events (including use of alcohol), and tempers increasing due to hot and humid weather, creating a dangerous combustible period. Summer, unless we live in an air-conditioned dwelling, necessitates that we get out onto the streets searching for cooling places, particularly in reaction to harsh winters. These public places and spaces are not necessarily safe, however (Delgado, 2024).

Grounding Chicago

Everyone seems to have an opinion on Chicago. That city, not surprisingly, has had extensive research on gun violence (Barnes, 2020). This is both good and not good from a public health standpoint. Readers have extensive material to select from depending upon interests. It signifies a city with limited safe harbors from this violence and in constant pain (trauma) of various types, with many of its neighborhoods bearing the scars of violence and corresponding trauma.

Urban funeral home gang shootings are not a new phenomenon that has emerged over the past few years. In 2015, Chicago funeral homes, for example, were put on heightened notice for gun violence (Jarrett, 2015), and that was 10 years ago! A decade is a long time in my book, so to speak! I noted earlier that I could have authored this entire book devoted to Chicago, and that says so much about how gun violence shapes life in this city's rough-and-tumble neighborhoods, reminding me so much about my youth in New York City's South Bronx, home to the nation's poorest congressional district then and still remains so today.

Case Illustration

Cities are the heart and soul of a nation, and that is a bias that I bring to this discussion of gun violence. Some cities are synonymous with shootings and gun deaths because of the extent and nature of shootings and the availability of major media outlets covering these stories and movies using these sites as a backdrop. No one city stands out. Thus, although a number of major cities receive attention in this book, Boston; Chicago; Detroit, Michigan; Washington, D.C.; Jacksonville; Miami, Florida; Oakland, California; Pittsburgh; Los Angeles, California; and New York, New York, find coverage of various depths throughout this book. Boston, Chicago, Jacksonville, and Pittsburgh, however, receive in-depth attention, with each having its own chapter, expanding the parameters of this phenomenon because it is a national public health problem.

It is no mistake that Chicago has been labeled the "mass shooting capital" of the U.S. (Adams, 2023), although other cities are not far behind. In Chicago, gun violence is not evenly spread out, which is certainly not unique to this city, with the south and west sides bearing the onus of this violence (Devaney, 2022). Highlighting one city allows readers to obtain a more in-depth portrait to emerge while still treating the problem of gun violence from a national viewpoint. This perspective also provides a more nuanced view to emerge, allowing a deeper understanding and appreciation of the consequences of gun violence on the death care system of that city.

Shootings at Funeral Homes

The funeral case illustration I selected was not Chicago's first funeral shooting. Two separate funeral home shootings almost 10 years apart illustrate how little gun violence has changed in this time period. Chicago funeral homes, which are often overlooked in any discussion of gun violence in this city, have had to struggle with this violence for almost one decade, far ahead of other communities confronting this form of violence and continuing to confront this violence in the present day (Jarret, 2015), as illustrated with the A.A. Rayner & Sons Funeral Home shooting:

> At A.A. Rayner & Sons funeral home in Chicago, Charles Childs is used to planning celebrations of long lives. His biggest concern traditionally has been timing the stop lights as he leads grieving families in a procession to the cemetery. These days, though, he has to worry about arranging a police presence to control the large, often emotional crowds that show up for the funeral… He used to see one or two violence-related funerals a year. Now, he says he directs one or two every month. So he has to take into consideration all sorts of things that he otherwise wouldn't—avoiding certain gang colors, navigating a tricky route between the service and the cemetery and hiring cops to keep the peace… At these funerals for interrupted lives, the mood is as much tense as somber. Eulogies must be delicately written for 'kids who may have been doing things they shouldn't have been doing,' Childs said. The smallest thing can turn grief to violence. 'It could be something so minor, like somebody stepping on somebody's foot or not saying hello or being asked to take their hat off'.

The funeral scene has taken on the semblance of an urban minefield, with life and death the outcome of successfully or unsuccessfully navigating it. Navigating this terrain of grief is arduous under most circumstances. However, doing so while dodging bullets and running for safety while screaming adds yet another dimension and challenge to the emotional and trauma-inducing experience of saying farewell to a loved one while trying to stay safe and alive (Ahlin, 2023).

Gun violence is not limited to any one neighborhood. However, its South Side stands out for attention historically and currently. Chicago's South Side is rightly considered "one of the major centers of African-American life in the United States with a legacy of accomplishment unparalleled in almost any other city in the country. Today, the South Side includes some of the most economically challenged neighborhoods in the United States" (Lowenstein & Hawarden, 2020, p.25). We must endeavor to not lose sight of numerous community assets, including small businesses and houses of worship, for example, which serve this community on a daily basis, while still keeping our focus on the outcomes of gun violence. I realize that is an arduous challenge, but one we must endeavor to confront and succeed at if communities are to have a chance at reaching their potential.

Gun violence in many of Chicago's low-resourced communities is often considered the major problem confronting residents, taking its place alongside drugs, particularly among youth, and we must not neglect the role police have played in these homicides, too (Hagan et al., 2022). A study of Chicago's Rosewood neighborhood, for example, found that 76% of its youth had witnessed gun violence in the previous year (Schober et al., 2024). Life expectancy differs significantly across neighborhoods, race, and socio-economic class. That is not an earth-shattering conclusion from a public health or social work standpoint, for example. Nevertheless, it is a stark reminder of how unfair life can be when based on an accident of birth.

Why the upsurge of shootings at funeral sites and last rites activities? These moments and places are where loved ones come to pay respect, love, and support each other. Nevertheless, there is no debating that these sacred moments and places have been severely compromised for a variety of reasons, particularly in urban centers with high gun and gang activities. The question remains, is it compromising in the immediate moment or for an extended period of time? If extended, for how long and how many life spans are altered?

Gangs play a key role in this upsurge in breaking cultural traditions, as in the case of Chicago (Goudie et al., 2023): "… dangerous and disrespectful funeral processions and out of control behavior at churches and burial sites have been going on for years, and sometimes the underlying motivation is old fashioned family squabbles, fueled by heartache and anguish. Chicago police and adjacent suburban departments trade intelligence cemeteries about upcoming funerals ripe for possible gang vengeance." Gangs, unfortunately, become an integral part of daily existence in some of this city's neighborhoods.

Development of a trusting working relationship between the police and cemeteries is a new dimension in police-community relations and one that warrants further exploration due to increases in violence at these sites. This necessitates the creation of various models to take into account local demographics and gun violence rates. In communities with high rates of gang violence, there has even been a call to have a special unit of the police department specifically devoted to working with funeral parlors to coordinate funeral processions.

This call can be a significant challenge in communities where there is a long history of distrust of the police, placing funeral establishments in a difficult situation of having to broker these two camps, so to speak. Pleasing a family's last wishes versus keeping attendees and staff safe may not represent much of a dilemma in some readers' minds. It does not take an active imagination to see how this struggle can exist and cause intense fears for safety in a neighborhood as violence spills over from last rites sites without regard to who is hurt.

Funeral shootings occur inside and outside of a funeral home, which may be a distinction without much of a difference. Nevertheless, physically entering a funeral home, in similar fashion to actually entering a house of worship, seeks to send a profoundly more powerful public message and act. It does not minimize a shooting at the front doorsteps. The same can be said about shootings outside of a cemetery versus going into this area. Entering a cemetery to commit a shooting brings a different level of mind-set and intent than waiting outside one to shoot at a parade of cars. A continuum of brazen acts at sacred sites brings an important viewpoint. Again, the case illustration is about Chicago. However, sadly, I could have selected from a range of cities.

As already noted, funeral shootings are certainly not unique to Chicago. A gunman shot and killed two people outside a Miami funeral being held for a shooting victim, for example, over 10 years ago (Reuters, 2012), illustrating this is now a modern phenomenon. Countless other examples have been cited throughout this book covering an extended period of time. The fallout on the funeral home is undeniable. Nevertheless, the following case illustration of Chicago's Weathersby drive-by (stolen car) funeral shooting encapsulates the significance of this phenomenon and why it is deserving of attention. On a 2020 hot and humid July day, a shooting transpired, spotlighting how the death care industry, in this instance a funeral home, has been changed in dramatic ways, including not being viewed as a sanctuary for grieving families.

Donnie Weathersby's funeral witnessed a high-casualty shooting with 15 wounded (10 females and 5 males, ages 21–65 years old), 9 seriously, with 2 eventually dying, giving the appearance of an urban war scene (Main & Charkes, 2020). Shots were returned by attendees, reinforcing the appearance of a war zone. The police were warned that a shooting would take place, and a patrol car was assigned to the site, but to no avail. Having a police presence, it bears noting, takes away from this solemn event, giving it more of a police state or war scene than a funeral scene.

Who was Donnie Weathersby? He was a 31-year-old Black-American resident of Chicago's South Side and gang member who was killed in a drive-by shooting. His funeral parlor shooting made national, if not international, news because of the number of causalities and the convergence of urban gun violence and a sacred/solemn moment considered to be safe from this form of violence, signaling a new "battlefront" for gun violence. Approximately 60 bullet shells were recovered at the scene, indicative of the carnage that transpired and giving the appearance of a battle scene.

When gun violence ensues at a funeral service causing casualties (physical/emotional injuries and even deaths), they are referred to as "second victims" or "co-victims," which can include faith-based leaders (Galiatsatos et al., 2021). Casualties can also occur as attendees scramble to seek safety and do not have to suffer a direct bullet wound. Mind you, attendee emotional damage escapes numeration, which is always challenging to count. This perennially seems to be the case, including discouraging future attendance at funerals for fear of gun violence when victim families need the emotional support the most. Failure to attend these ceremonies can cause family strains, too, because their absence is a public action that can be viewed as an insult to a family during an emotionally laden public event.

Family activism post-shootings has started to garner much-needed scholarly attention (Cook, 2020; Delgado, 2022), bringing a potential source of community activism with assistance from helping professions; this bodes well for the field, as taking a tragedy and converting it into positive change gives families an opportunity to direct their energies in an outward and healing manner. Activism brings hope while attracting others to the cause, which is good for mental health because group solidarity is affirming. Similar attention to the death care industry remains in its infancy at best, requiring attention, cultivation, resources, and a reconceptualization of how to support this field beyond its traditional boundaries. The attention to this industry has been primarily led by local media coverage, with scholarship far behind with notable exceptions.

Key Observations/Lessons

The implicit code widely shared that last rites are sacred moments should not be violated by gun violence, which has been the case for well over a decade. In late 2024, Chicago experienced another funeral-related shooting and death, illustrative of the key themes in this book (Johnson, 2024): "At 12:01 p.m., Dixmoor police were called to 147th Street and Seeley Avenue—where they found a white Jaguar sport-utility vehicle had crashed into a house, Dixmoor police Chief Lionel Smith said in a statement. Inside the vehicle, police found the woman who had been driving had suffered gunshot wounds. The woman had been part of a funeral procession that had just left St. Mark's Church in Harvey, police said. Turner was a sister and a mother—and to many, a well-known stylist. The funeral was for her brother, Chevelle Carter, who was shot and killed on Monday, Oct. 19, at 38th Street and Ellis Avenue in Chicago's Bronzeville neighborhood. A witness told police two gunmen got into a white vehicle and fled the scene after the shooting at 8:40 p.m. that evening. Some said late Saturday that the shooting was possible retaliation." A family is thus faced with two gun violence burials in the course of 2 weeks.

I wonder if I were to author this book 10 years from now how many funeral home shooting case illustrations I could draw upon. What can be done to prevent this tragedy from occurring again? I will focus my observations/lessons on law enforcement. What role can the police play to have a more active and effective role in preventing these types of shootings? Clearly, business as usual was not effective, necessitating a plan of action with a high probability of achieving success by more actively coordinating with communities.

For a police presence to be successful, there must be a close and trusting partnership between the death care sector and the police department based on mutual trust and willingness to collaborate without causing community backlash. This relationship, readers may not need reminding, must be based on mutual trust, requiring a plan based upon careful planning, wide community input, and monitoring. Mind you, having a police presence does not guarantee a safe final passage for a gun victim, as evidenced throughout the country.

Conclusion

Chicago is a beautiful and vibrant city with a rich history and home to countless immigrants and refugees, paralleling other older cities, particularly on the East Coast. If gun violence goes national in news coverage, it is very easy to get mired in crime, violence, death, and despair, shaping a national reputation. We must not forget that Chicago also harbors immense resources, dreams, and aspirations for a better future for children. However, guns have altered the character of many of its neighborhoods, leaving a lasting legacy and scar on the spaces and places stained by blood.

Funeral gun violence highlights how conventional barriers allowing grieving families to come together to support each other have been severely breached, leaving devastation at its door, and in the process altering business as usual when it comes to this sector. Communities cannot function without funeral homes. They are as consequential as any other organization in their midst, taking their place alongside other death care segments. How we protect attendees and staff is a priority for those in this industry if it hopes to make important advances in the future.

References

Adams, J. Q. A. (2023). *Examining the holistic health of urban African Americans experiencing continuous traumatic stress and gun violence in Chicago* (Doctoral dissertation, The University of North Carolina at Charlotte, N.C.).

Ahlin, E. M. (2023). *Violence in the heights: The torn social fabric of inner-city neighborhoods*. Routledge.

Barnes, P. (2020). *Living with killing: The lived experiences of young black men in South Chicago* (Doctoral dissertation, Walden University, Minneapolis, Minnesota).

CNN. (2024, July 8). *Chicago reels from violent holiday weekend: More than 100 shot, 19 fatally.* https://www.wpsdlocal6.com/news/chicago-reels-from-violent-holiday-weekend-more-than-100-shot-19-fatally/article_e7bce3f0-3d17-11ef-9e19-87f1ab6927e3.html

Cook, E. A. (2020). *Family activism in the aftermath of fatal violence*. Routledge.

Delgado, M. (2022). *The silent epidemic of gun injuries: Challenges and opportunities for treating and preventing gun injuries*. Oxford University Press.

Delgado, M. (2024). *Urban public spaces, events, and gun violence: Block parties, funerals, mother's day, and other community events*. Springer Publishers.

Devaney, K. (2022). *Death by Abandonment: Understanding North Lawndale's Historically High Homicide Rate* (Doctoral dissertation, University of Illinois at Chicago, Chicago, Il.).

Galiatsatos, P., Cudjoe, T. K., Bratcher, J., Heikkinen, P., Leaf, P., & Golden, S. H. (2021). Second victims: Aftermath of gun violence and faith-based responses. *Journal of Religion and Health, 60*, 1832–1838.

Goudie, C., Markoff, B., & Tresse, C. (2023, April 28). Violence continues to plague Chicago area funerals, including Friday's shooting in Maywood. *ABC7Chicago*. https://abc7chicago.com/chicago-funeral-violence-maywood-shooting-il-police/13193792/

Hagan, J., McCarthy, B., & Herda, D. (2022). *Chicago's reckoning: Racism, politics, and the deep history of policing in an American city*. Oxford University Press.

Hutchinson, B. (2023, August 21). 14-Year-old among 7 killed, 33 wounded in Chicago weekend gun violence. *ABC NEWS*. https://abcnews.go.com/US/14-year-7-killed-33-wounded-chicago-weekend/story?id=102422972

Jarrett, T. (2015, July 7). Chicago Funeral homes face challenges in gang territory. *NBC News*. https://www.nbcnews.com/storyline/chicagos-cruel-summer/chicago-funeral-homes-face-challenges-gang-territory-n386406

Johnson, D. (2024, November 2). Woman shot, killed in brother's funeral procession in South Chicago suburbs. *CBS*. https://www.cbsnews.com/chicago/news/woman-shot-killed-funeral-procession-south-chicago-suburbs/

Kotlowitz, A. (2020). *An American summer: Love and death in Chicago*. Anchor.

Lowenstein, J., & Dharmawardene, M. (2020). A violent thread: How violence cuts across the generations on Chicago's south side. In M. Siegler & S. Rogers Jr. (Eds.), *Violence, trauma, and trauma surgery* (pp. 25–50). Springer.

Main, F., & Charles, S. (2020, July 22). Gang feud mass shooting at South Side funeral home, sources say. *Chicago Sun Times*. https://chicago.suntimes.com/crime/2020/7/22/21334970/gang-feud-mass-shooting-funeral-home-auburn-gresham

Masterson, M. (2023, July 31). 5 people killed in shootings across Chicago over weekend: Police. *WTTW.Com*. https://news.wttw.com/2023/07/31/5-people-killed-shootings-across-chicago-over-weekend-police

Reeping, P. M., & Hemenway, D. (2020). The association between weather and the number of daily shootings in Chicago (2012–2016). *Injury Epidemiology, 7*, 1–8.

Reuters. (2012, March 31). Gunmen kill two outside Miami funeral of shooting victim. https://www.reuters.com/article/idUSBRE82U0GQ/

Schober, D. J., Wolf, A., Castro, M. C., Slezak, J., Hastings, P., & Latiker, D. (2024). An academic-community partnership to address gun violence in the Roseland Neighborhood of Chicago. *Family & Community Health, 47*(2), 141–150.

Seewer, J. (2024, July 3). Why mass shootings and violence increase during the summer. *AP News*. https://apnews.com/article/why-is-there-more-violence-summer-shootings-d5919ea324df5dbc732baf227123f849

Chapter 6
Boston, Massachusetts (Cemetery: Tombstone Destruction)

Introduction

I generally eschew uplifting Boston, Massachusetts, for attention in my writings, with few exceptions in the past. This book falls under that rare category of exceptions. I generally try to broaden the focus of my writings to other cities throughout the country, although always favoring large cities. I hope readers can see why I selected Boston by the end of this chapter. The convergence of multiple factors and events uplifted the focus of this chapter on cemeteries, a dimension that expands what it typically means to engage in gun violence in the death care sector.

Probably the most negative modern-day Boston image can be traced to the school busing episode that witnessed racial animosity and tensions during the early 1970s. Although the images portrayed by national media still linger in many people's eyes of school buses being confronted by crowds, it raised issues of racism that stained this city. However, what is little known is that Boston had a history of violence within its communities of color, with guns increasingly finding their way into settling disputes. Boston, like other cities, is experiencing a downward trend in gun violence rates. In 2023, there were 144 shooting victims, down 20% from 180 in 2022 and 52% from 277 in 2020 (Fortin, 2024). These shootings are ill-distributed across the city, not surprisingly. Neighborhoods such as Jamaica Plain, Roxbury, and Mattapan stand out disproportionately.

Grounding Boston

This chapter advances a different facet of urban gun violence in the death care sector and is a good follow-up to the funeral parlor case illustration on Chicago, Illinois, in the previous chapter (Chap. 5). Boston certainly has a national, if not

© The Author(s), under exclusive license to Springer Nature Switzerland AG 2025

M. Delgado, *The Death Care Industry and Urban Gun Violence*,
https://doi.org/10.1007/978-3-031-95682-9_6

international, reputation among those with interests in this nation's historical beginnings. This image has been carefully crafted and fostered. It may not surprise readers to know that there are neighborhoods where gun violence is fairly common, with other sections of the city oblivious to this violence and escaping its consequences. Boston, in all fairness, has not sat idly by, initiating community actions to stop gun violence, as readers will see.

Boston has the distinction of being home to many firsts in this nation's history due to its geographical location and access to the ocean. It is a city that brings many attributes, but it also has its share of urban ills and challenges, including gun violence. Thus, it is not surprising to see the emergence of coalitions of various types, including ones focused on gun violence and religious institutions.

Nuns Against Gun Violence, for example, has thrust Catholic nuns into advocates for gun violence prevention initiatives (Gallagher, 2024): "It is no surprise that in April 2023 Nuns Against Gun Violence was founded to bring together congregations of Catholic sisters to speak with a united voice against the crisis of gun violence. Sisters of St. Joseph of Boston have partnered with more than 60 communities who are involved in building this collaborative. They have also offered prayer services on Wear Orange Day, observed each year in early June. This event honors survivors and builds community with those working to end gun violence."

To be quite honest, I usually encounter priests at gun coalitions and as spokespersons for these efforts. Readers may have had different experiences. Involvement of the religious sector brings a level of "legitimacy," often moral in nature, as to why gun violence is a public health problem to communities and congregations, as witnessed with the historic Boston's Ten Point Coalition.

Boston's Ten Point Coalition (Berrien et al., 2021) was established in 2010, enlisting houses of worship as a key driving force behind this effort. It represented, arguably, a very different type of initiative in addressing gun violence, making it one of the earliest of such efforts. These types of undertakings embrace the "moral realities" of this violence and the political capital houses of worship and clergy bring that cross neighborhoods and traditional political discourse, which is essential in breaking down barriers on this significant public health problem. Business as usual can no longer be tolerated as a generation is essentially left to pick up the pieces, literally and figuratively, of this national public health problem.

One conversation I had with a religious leader raised a point that I have never heard before. Namely, once we have institutions normally not associated with gun violence entering this arena through coalition memberships and other high-profile activities, they essentially declare that they wish to take sides (Good Versus Evil), expecting retribution and no longer off-limits to gun violence. Of course, I also have heard the opposite when told that, in essence, when you attack church members and religious personnel, you are also attacking God and religion itself; this is a distinction without a difference as to who is off-limits to violence. Regardless of stance, for the gun violence field to succeed, it will have to expand its field of practice, opening up public spaces where violence can occur.

Boston, it may also be surprising, has a major memorial dedicated to Bostonians killed by gun violence, not uncommon in other cities with high gun violence histories. How big is Boston's gun violence problem? Well, big enough to have a major memorial dedicated to the victims! Boston's Gun Violence Memorial Exhibition, held by the Institute of Contemporary Art (ICA), sponsored a showing in 2024 (Institute for Contemporary Art, 2024):

> *The Gun Violence Memorial Project* creates space to gather and remember in light of the ongoing gun violence crisis. The memorial comprises four glass houses, each built of 700 clear bricks, a reference to the average number of gun deaths every week in the United States in 2019, when the memorial opened. The average number of U.S. weekly gun deaths in 2024 is 840. Many of the bricks hold remembrance objects—baby shoes, graduation tassels, and photographs—offered by families in honor of loved ones whose lives have been taken due to gun violence. These living memorials invite us to view the impact of gun violence through individual personal narratives.

There certainly are enough deaths to warrant a memorial project to signify a major gun violence problem for Boston, counter to possessing a national image of historical significance in this nation and an abundance of educational institutions of higher learning, shaping a well-crafted national and international reputation or image. The 2024 exhibition described above was sponsored by Boston's Institute for Contemporary Art attests to this acknowledgement.

All cities seem to have dual identities. One is positive and enjoys wide admiration, often reinforced through extensive and well-coordinated media campaigns intended to cultivate a well-polished view; the other can be negative and without the support of local and state government fostering this image and therefore subject to media accounts of news that brings the attention of a local audience. Boston has benefited from this campaign, making it an attractive city for tourists and corporate headquarters to relocate to, touting its attractive infrastructure, major transportation hub, and a wealth of intellectual brain power readily available. Its gun violence challenges, however, just do not make it to the national scene.

Case Illustration

The existence and meaning of a burial stone are not static, as noted by Cook (2011, p. 189): "The life of a funerary monument begins with a death; it is this ending that begins an existence of transformation, interaction, and experience. The identity commemorated, though not the individual, will continue to develop through the life of the material object." It makes sense that this viewpoint attracts actors and actions that can compromise the memory of the deceased, as illustrated in the Boston case through the vandalism of a headstone.

On March 27th, 2022, around 11 pm, a gang entered a local cemetery from the old Bromley Heath Projects in Jamaica Plain. They systematically knocked over the headstones of D'Andre King-Settles, Michael I. Ross, and John P. Cesar. These three victims had been shot to death, with King-Settles before he had turned 18. Not unexpectedly, less than 48 h later a rival gang knocked over the headstone of Gerrod Brown Jr., a 16-year-old victim of a gun shooting. Not only watching via Instagram the kicking down of King-Settles' headstone, but also witnessing spitting on it, serving as a triggering retaliatory act (Scott, 2022). Finally, they took his headstone and brought it back to the neighborhood (Cotter, 2022).

Word spread quickly on social media, further inflaming tensions between the two gangs. Police charged three teenagers with gravestone theft. How were the police able to quickly determine the culprits? All three teens were wearing court-mandated ankle bracelets from prior offenses, which made it easy to find them. A few days later, the police entered the graveyard, "closing in on a man who they said had been seen shortly beforehand with a gun. After a series of pat-frisks and minor tussles… officers found four guns, two on the backseat passengers and two in the car's glove compartment. Weapons charges ensued for the men, who police said had the guns illegally" (Cotter, 2022). It was obvious that the escalation of violence was imminent.

Cemetery manager Todd Burne noted as he assessed the damage: "'They don't really have respect for the people here,' Burne said. He said he's weighing security options, such as closing the gates at specific times and enforcing noise rules more stringently, though he doesn't want to keep people out who just want to come in and be respectful, so there's a balance. He doesn't want to tell the 'hundreds of mom and dads,' many working-class people of color from the surrounding neighborhoods that they can't come mourn when they wish" (Cotter, 2022).

Sadly, but not unexpectedly, a look at the birthdates of those buried there will find birthdays from the 1990s, 2000s, and 2010s. Celebrations honoring the dead do take place that can involve alcohol and other drugs, and encounters with other gangs can transpire, with corresponding violence occurring. Graveyard vandalism is an emerging phenomenon at this cemetery, as it is new across the country. Burne notes: "'It's just that they're getting caught more, maybe.' The walk around the graveyard passes by some of the headstones. King-Settles' is back up, as are Ross' and Cesar's. The police officers have hung onto Brown's after they retrieved it, leaving a gap in the line of headstones like a missing tooth. Burne shook his head again, and asked to no one in particular, 'Why can't you let them rest in peace.'" Sadly, this is not an uncommon question based upon my experience in the field.

It does not take great imagination to see how one act of vandalism escaped with the potential for serious gun violence that could result in more graveyards and heartbreaks, with corresponding death rites. Yes, no deaths did occur. Gun-related violence cannot be viewed solely from a bullets-fired standpoint. Escalation of violence can be the result of a perceived insult, following a path that continues further acts, eventually resulting in gun deaths and corresponding trauma for loved ones and their neighborhood.

Gun violence is often reported by the media by providing the immediate facts on the location of the shooting, victim characteristics, number and nature of casualties, and whether or not perpetrators were apprehended. However, the connective tissue, so to speak, of the background to this violence simply goes unnoticed and therefore unreported. This grounding necessitates coverage because it is part of the scene.

The aforementioned account of the life of a Boston cemetery, gangs, and gun violence grounds these shootings in the daily social fabric of community life and the lives of individuals who are gun and non-gun involved (Boston Herald, 2022). The aforementioned case illustration shows the nuances that are part of life and often overlooked in scholarly material. In this instance, it is part of a cemetery's history with gun violence, and a historical recorder for communities. Retribution and disrespecting a cemetery is a new dimension to a climate of violence that increasingly sees no boundaries.

Key Observations/Discussion

For some reason that I cannot identify at this point in time, I felt compelled to include Boston in this book. Mind you, Boston has a rich history and countless resources that make this city stand out. Nevertheless, it is a city with challenges that seem intractable, in similar fashion to the other cities discussed in this book. Boston's gun problem is not recent, as witnessed with the creation of the clergy 10-Point Coalition discussed earlier.

The gun problem is so formidable that it leaves Boston's streets and enters into its cemeteries. True, there was no gun shooting at this cemetery case illustration. However, the destruction of gravestones was an act of provocation that cannot be ignored and can spill over into other shooting galleries with resulting casualties of many different ages. Bullets do not discriminate as to who they strike and how they alter the history and character of the communities where they are commonplace. Cemetery violence, it also bears noting, does not have to encompass actual gunshots but it can certainly lead to it when retaliation ensues.

In March 2024, as a follow-up to this act of cemetery vandalism, indictments and criminal complaints were issued in federal court for over 40 individuals affiliated with the Heath Street Gang on racketeering conspiracy (O'Laughlin, 2024). The Homeland Security investigations caused the seizure of over 60 firearms used in an array of shootings, which also resulted in the shooting of a nine-year-old girl seriously wounded at a family gathering. The Heath Street Gang was also accused of drug trafficking and being part of a drug distribution network throughout Massachusetts, Maine, and California.

This Boston chapter was different from the ones on Chicago and Jacksonville because it spotlights two forms of violence on cemeteries. This illustration does not involve shootings, and readers may have initially questioned why include this chapter in this book. I hope they see the wisdom of expanding what gun violence entails. Violence, after all, can take various manifestations, compromising last rites ceremonies. These incidents, nevertheless, violate the sacredness of cemeteries and compromise communities.

Conclusion

Gun violence in its varied manifestations, including threats and mocking of victims, can bring consequences, both short- and long-term. The concept of community is not limited to the immediate geographical neighborhood and can extend to the local cemetery, a new dimension as to what constitutes being part of the neighborhood. I must admit that the local cemetery was never an extension of the "hood" when I was growing up in New York City.

Destroying tombstones may seem like a prank to some observers. No one is killed while this act is being perpetrated. In the case of Boston and other cities across the nation, it was not a prank and caused tremendous emotional pain and financial costs in rectifying this act. Further, and just as importantly, it left an indelible mark on the families by how their child's grave was disrespected, and the entire neighborhood knows this, which is the point of this action. A depressing message was sent to the community—there is no place to hide and escape the violence, emotional and/or physical! Simply stated, expect to live with despair!

References

Berrien, J., McRoberts, O., & Winship, C. (2021). Religion and the Boston miracle: The effect of black ministry on youth violence. In M. J. Bane (Ed.), *Who will provide? The changing role of religion in American social welfare* (pp. 266–285). Routledge.

Boston Herald. (2022, May 28). Boston cemetery grapples with uptick in gang activity. https://www.bostonherald.com/2022/05/28/boston-cemetery-grapples-with-uptick-in-gang-activity/

Cook, K. (2011). A different kind of afterlife: The cultural biography of headstones. In L. Amundsen-Meyer, N. Engel, & S. Pickering (Eds.), Identity crisis: Archaeological perspectives on social identity (pp. 189–198). Proceedings of the 42nd (2010) Annual Chacmool Archaeology Conference, University of Calgary, Calgary, AB.

Cotter, S. P. (2022, May 28). Boston cemetery grapples with 'uptick' in gang activity. *Boston Herald.* https://www.bostonherald.com/2022/05/28/boston-cemetery-grapples-with-uptick-in-gang-activity/

Fortin, M. (2024, January 10). Shootings in Boston reach historic low in 2023: 'It takes a lot of work'. *10 Boston.* https://www.nbcboston.com/news/local/shootings-in-boston-reach-historic-low-in-2023-it-takes-a-lot-of-work/3242768/

Gallagher, J. (2024, March 8). Sisters of St. Joseph of Boston partner with nuns against gun violence coalition. *The Pilot*. https://www.thebostonpilot.com/article.php?ID=196960#:~:text=Nuns%20Against%20Gun%20Violence%20is,changing%20needs%20of%20changing%20times

Institute for Contemporary Art. (2024). *The gun violence memorial project.* https://www.icaboston.org/articles/the-gun-violence-memorial-project-a-citywide-exhibition-and-living-memorial-to-victims-of-gun-violence-opens-in-boston-aug-29/%20https:/gunmemorial.org/MA/boston

O'Laughlin, F. (2024, February 14). 'Enough is enough': Gang terrorized Boston, bragged about murders, used kids as lookouts, feds say. *Boston 25.* https://www.boston25news.com/news/local/enough-is-enough-gang-terrorized-boston-bragged-about-murders-used-kids-lookouts-feds-say/GNBTNCS4LFABLJ54ZLRMMKZC5U

Scott, A. (2022). In a gang battlefield, no place to grieve. Long after murders, traumatized family and friends struggle to find help. *The Boston Globe*, pp. A1, A8.

Chapter 7
Pittsburgh, Pennsylvania's Destiny of Faith Church Shooting

Introduction

If one were to mention mass gun violence and Pittsburgh, Pennsylvania, it will have many of us thinking of the Tree of Life—Or L'Simcha Congregation shooting that occurred on October 27, 2018, when a gunman killed 11 and wounded 4, making national and international news (Oppenheimer, 2021). This chapter highlights another house of worship shooting that transpired in that city, but in a very different neighborhood and not as the result of racial hatred. The brazenness of the act did not make national, let alone international, news, but it sure sent shockwaves throughout Pittsburgh's surrounding communities. Pittsburgh can be considered a mid-size city, unlike the other cities highlighted in this book. Nevertheless, the challenges it faces with gun violence bring with them all of the characteristics and challenges that Boston, Massachusetts; Chicago, Illinois; and Jacksonville, Florida, face, and other cities, big, medium, and small, face.

Sadly, it is no secret that the targeting of houses of worship for violence is an age-old phenomenon. There are a series of shootings at houses of worship during funerals illustrative of this violence, displaying varying degrees of brazenness and a willingness to extract retribution on the part of shooters. These shootings publicly showed a total disregard for who is hurt in the process. These shootings have transpired within and outside of churches, broadening this sacred space. Big and small cities, too, have experienced these acts, uniting them in a club that no one wants to belong in, but one that is expanding in membership.

Houses of worship continue to exist in neighborhoods facing a host of social challenges, with gun violence being the latest in this long line of pain. They have been viewed as a sanctuary to turn to when facing many of life's most challenging times. Yes, they even exist in communities with high rates of violence, almost coexisting as places normally exempt from this violence. In addition, gun violence often

© The Author(s), under exclusive license to Springer Nature Switzerland AG 2025

M. Delgado, *The Death Care Industry and Urban Gun Violence*,
https://doi.org/10.1007/978-3-031-95682-9_7

exists in a whole range of spaces and places, but with rare exceptions, it does not find its way into a house of worship during a last rites ceremony.

As addressed earlier, houses of worship rarely witness gun violence, although there are several high-profile shootings that have shaken this institution at its roots, causing tremendous pain and soul-searching about our society, particularly our urban centers. It is because it is such a rare and egregious event that it generates extensive publicity and public reactions. The belief in this institution's sacredness has started to change causing houses of worship to close, with many of them in urban communities of color, bringing other challenges as to what will occupy their spaces (Delgado, 2025). This, too, is another form of death.

When gun violence does not respect the "House of the Lord," particularly during a last rites ceremony that is often viewed as a sacred moment for attendees, it shakes the foundation of a community, even those accustomed to having gun violence, as if any community can ever get used to such violence. That is what happened in Pittsburgh on a 2022 summer day, as detailed in the following case illustration. Unlike the Chicago case illustration, many individuals did not die or were wounded. Nevertheless, this does not diminish the impact of this act on the community.

Grounding Pittsburgh

Pittsburgh, in a similar fashion to other cities, has started to experience a decline in its gun violence, which must not be lost in reading this book. In 2015, it ranked as having the nation's 21st highest murder rate with 18.6 murders per 100,000. However, by 2022, it had declined to 12.3 per 1000, making it 58 among U.S. cities with a population of greater than 100,000 residents (Smith & Welch, 2023). Readers may rightly ask if this is the case, why include this city in this book? My intent is to show how gun violence, when grounded within different levels of intensity, is still a major public health problem, even in what can be considered a mid-sized city of 303,000, and one experiencing a pause in the growth of this form of violence.

The Pittsburgh illustration not only involved a shooting at a house of worship, but it was also not your "typical" drive-by associated with shootings. In fact, it involved two shooters that waited patiently for the service to be over and attendees leaving a church before starting their gunfire. Readers are reminded that shootings at houses of worship, funeral parlors, and cemeteries can transpire within and outside of these places, and that was the case in the Pittsburgh shooting.

It bears noting that an "atypical" drive-by is not exclusively a high-profile urban phenomenon. A drive-by shooting at the Living Water Baptist Church, High Point, North Carolina, with a population of 115,000 (36% Black), for example, had worshippers witnessing this violence during an open-door funeral that caused an 18-year-old to be killed and was widely attributed to gang retaliation (Smith, 2020). Open-door funerals can be held in a home or house of worship, weather permitting. Further, you do not need an invitation to attend and can typically just drop in to pay respects and stay as long as you wish.

Case Illustration

Pittsburgh has many of the factors we have become accustomed to seeing with urban gun violence (Wojciechowski, 2024). For example, it has a gun violence memorial that stands as a testament to this violence as a major problem (Taylor Jr., 2023):

> For the last two weeks, those that have stopped at the red light at Frankstown Avenue and N. Murtland Street in Homewood have seen the memorial. Filled with T-shirts of various colors, on each shirt is a name of a person, many of whom were Black-American, who died in this region to gun violence… Unfortunately, there are many more T-shirts, with the names of many more who have passed, way too soon. Heeding God's Call, along with Community and Family Builders, and Liddy Barlow of Christian Associates of Southwest Pa., have teamed up to create the gun violence memorial. A number of churches have been contacted throughout Pittsburgh to see which churches want to host the memorial on or near its grounds. In mid-May, the memorial was placed in a field next to Bethesda Community Church, in Homewood, along Bennett Street. On or near Mother's Day, the memorial was vandalized, T-shirts knocked off the small sticks and rebar of which they once rested.

Pittsburgh has a gun violence problem but is rarely included in the national litany of cities identified with this problem. This low profile was shattered when two gunmen entered a final rites ceremony at the Destiny of Faith Church (Brighton Heights neighborhood) with the primary intent of perpetrating harm regardless of who fell victim to their goals. The funeral service was for a victim killed 2 weeks earlier in a shootout between two neighborhood gangs.

This shooting was captured by surveillance cameras (Williams, 2022): "About an hour and a half into the service, a mourner—who was standing next to Hornezes' casket—was reading his obituary to the crowd and listing off the schools he attended when gunshots could be heard echoing in the church, the livestreamed footage shows. Masked mourners looked back toward the church entrance and hopped up from their seats, the video shows. A musician on stage huddled behind a wall, eyes wide with fear. 'What is happening?' a person could be heard saying amid the shouting and chaos before the video cuts off… Destiny of Faith Church." Surveillance cameras, it bears noting, did not deter this shooting.

The mass shooting caused five attendees to be injured by bullets, with a sixth victim injured while trying to escape the chaos. Three of the victims shot sought medical attention on their own, while emergency personnel transported the other three victims (Polina, 2022). Two adolescents (16- and 19-year-olds) were arrested. An estimated 20 rounds were fired during this gun episode. All attendees, including those leading the ceremony, also suffered. Rev. Brenda Gregg, the pastor at the Destiny of Faith Church, noted (Reardon, 2022): "This is probably, in my pastoral ministry that I have been doing over 30 years, this has been one of the most devastating days of my life, I would say," Mayor Gainey echoed this sentiment: "I never could have imagined it, that we would shoot up holy ground."

Although a police presence was requested for fears of potential retaliation, none were assigned, raising questions of how decisions to make them available when requested are granted. A surveillance camera was located outside and near the church, with the shooting captured on tape and used as evidence at trial. There were fears of violence at this funeral. Police were not provided, raising serious issues about safety protocols (Valente, 2022) and illustrating how fear or terror can quickly spread throughout a community.

We usually think about a shooting at a house of worship as only having an impact at the shooting site, which is significant enough. However, as in the case of Pittsburgh, the shooting caused a ripple effect, impacting the neighborhood and nearby churches. Of course, it would not be a stretch to think of similar consequences of shootings at the other "sacred" sites focused on in this book. Nevertheless, these reactions were not covered by the media.

Key Observations/Lessons

Pittsburgh witnessed a shooting that started in a church but continued outside as the gunmen fled, expanding the terror terrain and radiating out into other public spaces. Rev. Gregg's glimpse into the trauma this shooting caused her and service attendees, too. "Recovering" from this experience, if that is ever possible, takes time, help, resources, and patience. Equally important is that a sacred space was violated with impunity, legitimizing this site as a target. These spaces meet a wide range of needs in a community and are compromised to the point where attendees may be reluctant to continue attending in the future, further isolating them from the broader community.

Many aspects emerge in reviewing the Pittsburgh church shooting, which, in many ways, was not totally unexpected by the Church and attendees, which is not untypical. Mind you, it does not make the shooting any easier to digest. Harm was not just perpetrated on attendees paying their final respects. The harm radiated in the neighborhood. The fact that it was videotaped did not deter the shooters, who acted with impunity, raising questions about this strategy of ensuring safety for attendees.

A police presence, to be quite honest, does deter shootings at death care events, as to be expected. However, the police in this instance did not take the request for their presence seriously, which possibly could have averted a shooting. Their presence, as in Chap. 5's discussion of Chicago's case illustration, did not stop the mass shooting there! There is a need for a protocol that has a high probability of deterring shootings, which requires a high degree of coordination and deployment of resources. Further research is called for in order to shape interventions that increase the likelihood of success.

Conclusion

The Pittsburgh illustration showed the brazenness of the act and how perpetrators waited patiently inside of the church for the right moment to do their shooting. The fact that surveillance equipment was present and captured the shooting, which was widely disseminated, did not deter the shooting. This raises questions on the deliberations covered in this book on how surveillance equipment can deter gun violence and the costs of installing and maintaining this equipment. This focus may serve to give a false sense of security.

Readers are well positioned for the final case illustration focused on cemetery violence, not with the use of gunfire but with the use of social media to insult the buried and send a message to the broader community in the process. This final case illustration positions readers well for the final section and a focus on research, education, and practice recommendations. Business as usual regarding death care shootings and other forms of violence necessitates research, innovative thinking, and actions to increase the chances of achieving much-needed success.

References

Delgado, M. (2025). *When the Lord's House closes: Church closings and urban community practice*. Oxford University Press.

Oppenheimer, M. (2021). *Squirrel hill: The tree of life Synagogue shooting and the soul of a neighborhood*. Knopf.

Polina, R. (2022, October 29). 2 arrests linked to shooting outside Pittsburgh church during funeral service. *New York Post*. https://nypost.com/2022/10/29/2-arrests-made-in-pittsburgh-in-connection-to-the-destiny-of-faith-church-shooting/

Reardon, S. (2022, October 29). 6 injured in "targeted shooting" outside Pittsburgh church during funeral, 2 arrested. *CBS News*. https://www.cbsnews.com/news/pittsburgh-funeral-shooting-6-hurt-2-teens-arrested/

Smith, A, (2020, November 19). Gangs believed to be involved in deadly shooting at High Point Church. *MYFox8.Com*. https://myfox8.com/news/gangs-believed-to-be-involved-in-deadly-shooting-at-high-point-church/

Smith, R. D., & Welch, J. C. (2023). Seeking the peace: Anti-gun violence cadres, concepts, and connections in Pittsburgh. *Society, 60*(1), 54–67.

Taylor, Jr. R. (2023, June 9). 'A reminder that people do care.' Gun violence memorial in Homewood honors the lives lost. *Pittsburgh Courier*. https://newpittsburghcourier.com/2023/06/09/a--reminder-that-people-do-care-gun-violence-memorial-in-homewood-honors-the-lives-lost/

Valente, M. (2022). 'Continued shock': Priest of nearby church reacts to Destiny of Faith church. *4ABC*. https://www.wtae.com/article/continued-shock-priest-of-nearby-church-reacts-to-destiny-of-faith-church/41810454

Williams, A. R. (2022, October 28). Pittsburgh police say 6 shot in church during funeral service. *USA Today*. https://www.usatoday.com/story/news/nation/2022/10/28/pittsburgh-police-say-6- shot-church-during-funeral-service/10625241002/

Wojciechowski, T. (2024). Neighborhood disorder as a predictor of perceptions of firearm access: Examining peers effects. *Injury, 111701*.

Chapter 8
Jacksonville, Florida (Cemetery Violence and Social Media)

Introduction

This final case illustration pushes the conventional boundaries of how we typically think about urban gun violence. As already noted, I originally was planning on only using three case illustrations, with the original list being Boston, Massachusetts (Cemetery Vandalism of Graves); Chicago, Illinois (Funeral Parlor Shooting); and Pittsburgh, Pennsylvania (Church Shooting). As this book unfolded and gun violence and its varied manifestations emerged in saliency, it introduced an opportunity to broaden the field on what constitutes gun violence and its consequences and is reflective of how violence can be perpetrated after a final rites event, with even more potential deadly repercussions following.

Some readers may argue that including a chapter on "gun violence" that does not actually involve gunshots may be a "stretch." We must eschew concrete thinking on a subject that brings both physical and broad emotional manifestations. The existence of gang graffiti serves multiple goals beyond marking territories (Hughes et al., 2021), is no longer limited to neighborhood walls, and has crept into cemeteries, bringing along gun violence.

Stylianou-Lambert and Widmaier (2023) offer a historical perspective on death and photography that helps ground our modern-day experiences: "Photography has been associated with death and used for mourning practices since its inception. The invention of photography had a profound influence on how people remember and mourn the dead. Nowadays, the constant availability of mobile phone cameras, digital networks, social platforms, and new printing technologies have changed the kinds of photographs which are taken and how they are shared and displayed."

Digital selfies taken at places of profound pain and suffering, as in the case of Auschwitz and other Holocaust-related sites, for example, raise important ethical considerations on how places and spaces can be purposefully or innocently compromised (Hodalska, 2017; Zalewska, 2017). Digital photographs can serve to empower

© The Author(s), under exclusive license to Springer Nature Switzerland AG 2025

M. Delgado, *The Death Care Industry and Urban Gun Violence*,
https://doi.org/10.1007/978-3-031-95682-9_8

mourners through the level of detail they can reveal (Widmaier, 2023); they can also seriously compromise the mental health of mourners when used to insult the deceased as in the case of this Jacksonville, Florida, case illustration.

The digital nature of these photographs lends itself to wide distribution, helping recipients to address pain, mourn, or celebrate the life of the deceased depending upon goals (Santi & Bianchi, 2023, p.1): "With the advent of the digital age, we are witnessing a revolution in space and in the way in which everyday life and, also, the end of life is faced, to the point that physical death no longer coincides with digital death, allowing, the permanence of the individual in the virtual space."

Gun violence can manifest itself in many different forms and may even not involve actual shootings. Violence, we must not forget, can be both physical and psychological. These two forms, of course, can involve both, as experienced in Philadelphia, for example. The convergence of gun violence and social media is a deadly combination that can carry over to cemeteries (Gore, 2024):

> A well-known figure in Philadelphia's bustling hip-hop scene, rapper YBC Dul had a following many musicians would envy. He had more than 30,000 monthly listeners on Spotify, and his YouTube and Instagram videos drew more than a million views. But some of those posts showed Dul's exploits as a reputed criminal gang leader—videos he shot and uploaded to social media himself. In February, police say, he recorded his most brazen act: digging up the grave of a murdered gang rival, then taunting the dead man's crew by posting the video online. Days later, Young Bag Chaser Dul—real name, Abdul Vicks, age 25—was gunned down in broad daylight on a busy downtown street… From New York to Chicago to Los Angeles, experts say, cases like Vicks' are playing out in cities nationwide, with rivalries or personal beefs being turbocharged in cyberspace.

It bears noting that the influence of social media in fostering gun violence is greatly underrated and therefore under-researched. Selfies and death, it bears noting, can be viewed as "Post-Modem Photography," introducing a new form of photography, with a backdrop that enhances the image. When selfies are casted as a backdrop (context), making the setting a critical element in the storytelling, an "afterlife," so to speak. This design concept has evolved to become an integral part of an attempt at perpetrating harm. The challenge that the Jacksonville case illustration presents is not unique to that city. It is possible to create fear without having to use a gun and firing bullets. Psychological acts are a form of terror and evident in this final case illustration!

Grounding Jacksonville

The filming of a video for dissemination on social media, as an act of violence, was too important not to spotlight, introducing this act to readers and the field. I undertook an extensive literature review and could not find a single scholarly article on undertaking a music video as an act of violence at a gun victim's grave. "Soiling the grave of a deceased person," in all likelihood a former gang member, seems to be an emerging field of study and practice. It brings the potential for further retributive violence, including the use of guns.

When one thinks of Florida, two cities seem to come to mind for most readers—Miami and Orlando. These cities have a tremendous draw on a national and international level. Jacksonville, in the northern part of the state, does not seem to draw much attention. That, of course, is one person's assessment, although Jacksonville can be considered by most reader's standards as a "big" city, with a population of almost 1 million residents, having a major airport, and in a state that has a national profile. Thus, in all honesty, it is not a city that gets major national coverage of gun violence, although this issue is clearly a major public health problem in that city's communities of color. Jacksonville has been referred to as the "Murder Capital of Florida."

I have visited Jacksonville about half a dozen times, and it's a city that I write about in this book that I am least familiar with, but I thought it was important to include because it typifies how most cities with large populations of people of color are experiencing gun violence. Jacksonville had over 160 shootings in 2023 (Brooks, 2024), over 3 per week, making this issue salient for the overall community but particularly in its neighborhoods of color. Almost 94% of those killed were Black American males, with over half of the victims under the age of 30. More broadly, this city ranked 23rd in highest murder rate out of the 75 largest cities in the country. As of December 13, 2023, there had been 28 mass shootings in Florida, injuring 127 people and killing 36.

In this case illustration, readers will see the violation of what is widely considered a sacred space at a deep moment of sadness, but not using guns or even threatening to use them to inflict harm. The "incident" addressed in this chapter, by the way, is experienced in other locales across the country and is not unique to this city.

The saying "Justice delayed is justice denied" comes to mind. Early in this book, the topic of finding justice in the criminal justice system for murders was raised and how low clearance rates have made believing in the justice system difficult in the case of Nixon, a mother of a gun victim (Burgess, 2024): "On the five-year anniversary of her son's death, Nixon still has no answers. She said she's noticed an increase in gun violence in her hometown of Jacksonville. 'It's sad, it's very heartbreaking,' she said, 'We're burying our kids. If you live to be 18 in our community it's a blessing. My son reached 18½ and then his life was taken.'"

There is no question that law enforcement agents' presumptions of who deserves homicide loss survivor of governmental resources, responsiveness, and other types of support is considered worthy or unworthy and wields great influence on how a community views them (Wesely & Dewey, 2024). This stance, however, carries over into other spheres, including institutional commitment to solve crimes such as murder. When we cannot count on law enforcement and the legal system to achieve justice, then it falls into the hands of those who have been aggrieved to achieve it. From a community standpoint, which is dangerous!

It was important in conceptualizing this chapter that we expand our vision of gun violence and how an initial act that led to a murder can be further exacerbated by violent acts that seek to soil or destroy the memory of the deceased, in similar fashion to the Boston case illustration in Chap. 5. The focus on a "different" form of violence, I believe, broadens the picture to be more representative of how gun violence can assume many different forms and challenges the field of gun violence to broaden its conception of violence.

Gun violence at sacred places has evolved as this form of violence and gained currency in the nation's urban centers. Retribution, as in this case illustration, has historically been a key motivator for extracting deadly revenge, with guns gaining in prominence as the weapon of choice. Defining violence as needing to involve actual shootings is too narrow a focus, as discussed in this chapter on a Jacksonville cemetery.

This final case illustration shows how using guns as a symbol, or prop, can be considered an act of violence without firing a single bullet! This act can cause great emotional harm to loved ones thinking that their deceased relative or friend is in their final resting place and at peace. Social media has changed in this age of gun violence, broadening the intended audience beyond the immediate victim and their loved ones in attendance.

Some astute readers may say that social media has evolved over the past several decades and become the "gang graffiti of the 1980s" (Williams, 2021), with all of its intents and, unfortunately, even more deadly consequences. Walls were the writing tablets for graffiti during this early period. Defacing these walls was considered an act of aggression with potentially deadly results. The messages conveyed through social media are much more elaborate and easily spread, bringing a greater potential to stir violence that can, in turn, cause greater use of guns. Using the graves of the "enemy" as a prop only intensifies the emotional reactions of those they are intending to disrespect.

There is general agreement that most gang social media challenges remain as such and do not result in violence. However, some, particularly those that are extraordinarily egregious, can result in violent retaliation. Not with a countering social media message, but with actual gun violence. Murals have been used in the past to memorialize dead gang members, among others, replacing having to attend a cemetery to pay respects to the deceased, which was expensive and time-consuming because of travel distances.

I have attributed their origins and popularity to the role that murals historically played in the Caribbean and Latin America, and transported to this country through migration. This graffiti has been called "graffiti of grief" (Lübbers, 2007). Defacing these murals was intended and viewed as an act of provocation, with a very high likelihood of escalating into physical violence. The greater availability of guns, particularly high-powered ones, has made the potential of this escalation more deadly and memorable.

"Metastasizing disrespect" is a graphic term for capturing how social media inflames potentially dangerous situations that can often lead to gun violence (Szabo, 2023). I think it portrays how the climate of violence has changed and spread, giving new meaning to the terms "climate change" or "ominous cloud." One police chief (Michel Moore, Los Angeles) noted: "'What used to be communicated on the street or in graffiti or tagging or rumors from one person to another, it's now being distributed and amplified on social media,' he said. 'It's meant to embarrass and humiliate others.'" Allowing these acts of aggression to go unanswered tarnishes the reputation of the intended target in a highly public manner.

Using social media to post a video disrespecting a grave can be viewed as an evolution of violence because of its increased potential for causing physical injuries and even further deaths, particularly if those related to the deceased seek retribution. Social media has the potential to reach a broad audience, unlike murals that only limit their exposure to those physically present. Thus, disrespecting someone, often the case involving a gang member, can even have an international audience, adding further insult to this act of violence! Readers are well positioned to read the following Jacksonville case illustration, which expands how we view and interpret an act of violence at what many consider a sacred site.

Case Illustration

Cemeteries can serve as a backdrop for films, with horror movies standing out, and now more recently as scenes for rap videos honoring dead gang members and disseminated on social media. A brief historical review is in order. Hip-hop marked a major milestone when it celebrated its 50th anniversary in 2023. Hip-hop is anything but simple. One dimension is a subgenre called "drill rap," which emerged in the 2010s in Chicago's mean streets drawing inspiration from drug culture, guns, and gang violence, and widely witnessed in Jacksonville, FL. This music celebrates murders of gang rivals or what is referred to as "oops" in music videos and social media, intending to be confrontational and romanticize extreme violence. Hall et al. (2022) note that advocates of this music reflect the realities of day-to-day life in high-violence environments.

Jacksonville has multiple gangs, not surprisingly, with two seemingly standing out because of their particular hatred of each other, which increases the likelihood of violence begetting even greater violence (First Coast News, 2024):

> The 45th Street area of the city is home to one of the most well-known groups called 6-block made famous by Foolio, one of the area's most popular rappers, whose real name is Charles Jones. Some younger gang members affiliated with 6-block call themselves Bully Gang. Most members of Bully Gang are associated with Foolio. During the last few years, Jacksonville has received a lot of media attention nationwide from Foolio's beef with Yungeen Ace, another famous Jacksonville rapper… Ace is a member of a gang called ATK, which Jacksonville police have said stands for "Ace's Top Killers." Many members of ATK also claim a gang called NHG, which stands for No Hospital Gang. NHG and ATK are also closely aligned with a set called Backstreet.

A highly well-publicized incident can cause an abrupt and deadly gun violence episode, with a graveyard serving as a backdrop for violence. Although countless numbers of gang members had been arrested over the last several years, this has not slowed the escalation of gun violence, as evidenced in the Jacksonville cemetery case illustration (First Coast News, 2024):

> About seven months ago, Foolio and members of Bully Gang and 6-Block went to a cemetery to film a music video for Jake Jhitt, a Bully Gang rapper whose real name is Jayquan Pickens. While there, the group posed for photos in front of the burial site of Royale De'Von Smith Jr., whose nickname was 23. Smith, 18, was in a car with best friend Yungeen Ace and two other teens in June 2018 celebrating Smith's birthday at a restaurant at the St. Johns Town Center. As they were driving away from the area, their car was riddled with bullets killing Smith and two other men including Ace's brother. Ace was the only survivor.

Much to no one's surprise, no arrests resulted, further adding insult to the sorrow experienced by his loved ones even when there was no mystery as to the culprits. The slogan "No justice, no peace" comes to mind. This highlighted an experience of other cities across the nation when families of victims cannot find justice because of a lack of an arrest and subsequent trial (PthugginTV, n.d.):

> 6-Block members were reportedly responsible for the shooting. Several of the people in the photos at Smith's grave held their shoes up to Smith's grave marker. Some held up their middle fingers while others formed their hands into the shape of guns or gang signs. Soon after the photos were posted, ATK and NHG members took to social media and vowed payback.

Details on the Murder of BG Ybezzy (PthugginTV, n.d.):

> Around 9:40 p.m. on May 17, a Bully Gang member who rapped under the name BG Ybezzy ... was killed in Jacksonville's Moncrief Park area... When officers arrived, they found two boys and one adult male ... suffering life-threatening injuries. BG Ybezy, whose real name is Adrian McKinzie, 16, was rushed to the hospital where he was pronounced dead.

It bears noting that McKinzie's family member (woman) was shot where he had been killed when holding a memorial in his honor, illustrating how there is no limit to the misery and despair that a ceremony honoring a victim of gun violence. The ceremony, it bears noting, entailed releasing balloons to honor the deceased. Paying tribute was not meant to disrespect anyone!

Key Observations/Lessons

Providing a context for cemetery shootings was extremely important to ground these events, helping us better understand the history and convergence of numerous factors to create a highly combustible shooting scene. The emergence of urban music videos and violence as a backdrop to gun violence without regard to scene and context, with guns as a vehicle for settling disputes and enhancing reputations, introduces a Brave New World to the gun violence field.

Music is not new to funerals and is integral to the urban music scene, including the glorification of gun violence! Using cemeteries as a backdrop to perpetrate revenge brings a new dimension to understanding gun violence at these sites. Social media can be an effective tool in helping people and communities come together and heal. Clearly, the scenario described above presents a new dimension to what it means to mourn or celebrate a life cut short by gun violence. Cemeteries are places to express sorrow as well as celebrate a life, sharing with the deceased our happiness and wishes. Violating these scared spaces takes on added significance as a result. Readers, of course, can make up their own minds. The picture of cemeteries is far more complex, with social media adding new perspectives, either positive or negative, as found throughout this book.

Conclusion

I hope that readers see the wisdom of adding this chapter on Jacksonville, social media, gangs, gun violence, and cemeteries. Guns are not only instruments of pain and potential death but can also be instruments to inflict psychic pain and suffering on families and loved ones. Readers would agree that an individual waving a gun around in public, even if it is not loaded, is an act of violence. Social media, too, can be a form of violence for a family and others in great emotional pain.

This book spotlighted several major urban centers, although funeral-related shootings are a national phenomenon involving medium-sized and smaller cities, too, and community-centered. Size does matter in the amount and nature of resources that can be made available when needed, particularly during an emergency such as an unexpected gun shooting involving multiple victims at a solemn event. It is not a leap to say that major urban centers are disproportionately represented in these shootings, particularly in the case of youth, young adults, and communities of color. The ramifications of this generational public health epidemic will be felt well into the future of these communities, cities, and nation, as significant segments are lost along with their creativity, energy, and potential contributions to their community and the nation.

Last rites are sacred moments and ceremonies that leave positive or negative lasting impressions depending on how they transpire. These moments, in turn, can be severely compromised when acts of violence are perpetrated. Use of social media as a weapon to soil a grave and the memory of the deceased can be very psychologically violent and destructive, bringing many of the same goals when guns are used to hurt people, families, and, for that matter, communities, too. I have yet to encounter a gun shooting involving a baby's baptism, but it is just a question of time, I am sorry to say. Shootings at adult baptisms are not uncommon, however (Gaston Gazette, 2022).

Although Jacksonville was the backdrop for this chapter, social media finds its way into countless other communities, perpetrating pain and anger regardless of setting and circumstances. Cemeteries must never be viewed as plots for storytelling, no pun intended. That applies to Hollywood and home movies alike. These media efforts can lead to real-life deaths and injuries for those "lucky" enough to survive to tell the tale.

Part II provided a more detailed examination of a geographical entity and how gun violence at events shares much in common but also brings unique circumstances to account for the final rites, occasion, and locale. Themes cross funeral homes, cemeteries, and houses of worship, and also bring unique aspects for designing interventions. This book used four urban case illustrations to tell the stories: (1) Chicago (funeral home shootings) (Chap. 5); (2) Pittsburgh (house of worship) (Chap. 7); (3) Boston (cemetery—destroying gravestones) (Chap. 6); and (4) Jacksonville (cemetery—social media use of a grave as an insult), highlighting the three domains of the death scenes. Each city highlighted a particular aspect of the death scene, allowing readers to appreciate the uniqueness of these sites, uplifting the role of context, and informing education, research, and practice.

References

Brooks, N. (2024, April 29). Ex-gang member pledges to end gun violence in his Jacksonville community. *ACTIONNEWSJAX*. https://www.actionnewsjax.com/news/local/ex-gang-member-pledges-end-gun-violence-his-jacksonville-community/E5K2YMJICBHVHOZ6DDDDNPEMWM/

Burgess, C. (2024, June 25). Jacksonville mom calls end of gun violence on the anniversary of her son's death. *First Coast News.Com*. https://www.firstcoastnews.com/article/news/local/jacksonville-mom-calls-end-gun-violence-on-the-anniversary-of-her-sons-death/77-fc8985f2-eac6-4d63-9133-577225c1344c

First Coast News. (2024, January 30). *Drillin' & killin' | Jacksonville's deadly gang beef takes disturbing twist in graveyard*. https://www.firstcoastnews.com/article/news/crime/jacksonville-rappers-drill- eef-foolio-yungeen-ace-tillie-rico-osama-jake-jhitt-bully-gang-atk-6block-kshordy-spinabenz-whoppa-wit-da-choppa-nhg/77-2fcb17d0-d408-472c-a79e-9668f63d0283

Gaston Gazette. (2022, March 30). *Gun violence victim Johnny 'John Luke' Moore at his baptism*. https://www.gastongazette.com/videos/news/2022/03/30/gun-violence-victim-johnny-john-luke-moore-barber-baptism-video/7222971001/

Gore, J. P. (2024, September 19). How social media turbocharges gun violence. *Word in Black*. https://wordinblack.com/2024/09/how-social-media-turbocharges-gun-violence/

Hall, B., Khan, R., & Eslea, M. (2022). Criminalising black trauma: Grime and drill lyrics as a form of ethnographic data to understand "gangs" and serious youth violence. *Genealogy, 7*(1), 2.

Hodalska, M. (2017). Selfies at horror sites: Dark tourism, ghoulish souvenirs and digital narcissism. *Zeszyty Prasoznawcze, 2*(230), 405–423.

Hughes, L. A., Schaible, L. M., & Kephart, T. (2021). Gang graffiti, group process, and gang violence. *Journal of Quantitative Criminology, 38*, 365–384.

Lübbers, G. (2007). The graffiti of grief: Violence, death and remembrance in Pittsburgh gang neighborhoods. *Paideuma*, 145–160.

PthugginTV. (n.d.). *ATK/ NHG VS 6 Block/ Bully Gang: Jacksonville's Duval County Never Ending Gang War!* https://www.youtube.com/watch?v=w6kIAht-hbQ

Santi, F., & Bianchi, D. (2023). Bereavement in the digital age: The challenges of online sharing and digital memory preservation. *Medicina, 7*(2), e2023023.

Stylianou-Lambert, T., & Widmaier, L. (2023). Everyday photography and mourning in the 21st century. *Photographies, 16*(1), 3–18.

Szabo, L. (2023, August 31). 'All we want is revenge': How social media fuels gun violence among teens. *CNN*. https://www.cnn.com/2023/08/31/health/social-media-gun-violence-kff-health-news-partner/index.html

Wesely, J. K., & Dewey, S. (2024). "I Want That Money Saved for 'Real' Victims": Homicide detectives' perceptions of victims and impacts on advocacy and services for loss survivors. *Homicide Studies, 28*(2), 220–244.

Widmaier, L. (2023). Digital photographic legacies, mourning, and remembrance: Looking through the eyes of the deceased. *Photographies, 16*(1), 19–48.

Williams, M. (2021, April 26). Rival Jacksonville gangs locked in deadly battle glorified in new viral rap music videos. *First Coast News*. https://www.firstcoastnews.com/article/entertainment/music/yungeen-ace-julio-foolio-jacksonville-rappers-rival-groups-atk-kta-in-deadly-beef-who-i-smoke-when-i-see-you/77-6d993faa-b014-4d8c-99be-de8d9fcdb948

Zalewska, M. (2017). Selfies from Auschwitz: Rethinking the relationship between spaces of memory and places of commemoration in the digital age. *Studies in Russian, Eurasian and Central European New Media, 18*(1), 95–116.

Part III
Research, Education, and Practice

Chapter 9
Research

Introduction

This chapter is the first of three chapters on how research, education, and practice can help bridge the lacuna between the academic world and the "real world." One of these realms cannot succeed without the other two realms, making a comprehensive approach arduous but extremely important to achieve. Thus, it is appropriate to start this final section of the book with the importance of research in shaping our thinking and actions on gun violence's reach into the death care sector and how best to address this growing form of violence. Research translation on gun violence, however, brings considerable challenges (Noorman et al., 2025), which can be expected to increase in significance when entering into what are considered new neighborhood terrains, such as the death care sector.

There certainly is a great deal for us to learn about this vital segment of society as it relates to gun violence. Brandolino et al. (2024), for example, concluded based on their research that outpatient models for firearm-related injuries and trauma care are not only inconsistent but unstandardized across trauma centers, compromising our understanding of how gun violence undermines health. Research strategies are welcomed by those in the gun violence field. We often hear that education is a lifelong process or journey involving a multitude of approaches, some formal and many informal. Research, however, uplifts those in this sector, which is an important place to begin in the crafting of urban interventions for the death care sector.

Let's face it, we cannot make significant inroads into gun violence and the death care industry, or any other arena, without research guiding our decision-making on best approaches. This section is arduous to write because of the paucity of research and the resulting tremendous gaps in knowledge that currently exists. In other words, "any research is better than no research." Lack of funding in this arena means that we must prioritize areas for future research considering different urban centers,

© The Author(s), under exclusive license to Springer Nature Switzerland AG 2025

M. Delgado, *The Death Care Industry and Urban Gun Violence*,
https://doi.org/10.1007/978-3-031-95682-9_9

avoiding a focus exclusively on large cities frequently highlighted in the national media.

The first or foundational step is to obtain a grasp of the extent of the problem, and this calls for establishing some form of foundation or baseline. For example, there is a loud call for improving systematic data collection to track police violence toward youth (Oppenheim et al., 2024). There is no question that cemetery and funeral home shootings are a national problem increasing in significance. To what extent remains an unanswerable question and will remain so without national leadership answering this question based on research that can establish baselines, with results easily retrievable for developing interventions.

Academics bring scholarly credentials to the topic of gun violence, and that knowledge must not be minimized. However, there is no substitute for lived experience in helping us discover, or "unlocking" solutions with a high likelihood of success (Dillard et al., 2023). The death care sector bears witness to how gun violence has shaped family and neighborhood dynamics during particularly trying times, with lessons learned through these insights shaping initiatives with a high likelihood of achieving success. This calls for major urban research undertakings to tap their voices in shaping how we respond to their unique needs.

Community-based participatory action research, for example, is so much more than a research approach. It has the potential to be a liberating tool (Malone et al., 2024, p. 901) for urban communities of color addressing gun violence in their midst to "equip credible and trustworthy community members with mental health knowledge and skills to support other community members experiencing mental health challenges." Research can be a form of intervention while in the process of creating knowledge.

Readers, from a research standpoint, should not be surprised by my call for a systematic self-reporting system on gun violence, and more specifically, gang-related funeral processions, as noted by a local sheriff in Illinois (Inklebarger, 2018): "It's been a challenge to understand the scope of the problem, he said, adding, 'There isn't necessarily a funeral-related or a death care industry-related code that we can just stick into a computer and have it spit back out how many incidents we've had.'" Understanding the extent of gun shootings within the death care sector will help us comprehend the extent and varied manifestations of this public health problem.

Bancalari et al.'s (2022) review of youth exposure studies of endemic community gun violence identified five themes illustrating the challenges that the field faces in crafting interventions: "(1) a lack of consensus regarding the range of experiences that constitute community gun violence, (2) exposure to violence involving a firearm as distinct from that with other weapons, (3) a need to conceptualize multiple dimensions of gun violence exposure, (4) differential impacts of exposure to community gun violence across developmental stages, and (5) how indirect gun violence exposure uniquely contributes to cycles of community violence."

Further, how can we logically make sense of gang homicides, for instance, as a backdrop to gun violence at a last rites ceremony (Urbanik & Roks, 2021)? First of all, we must make note that no two contexts are similar, requiring us to pause and differentiate from general approaches and overviews. This is not to say that important information cannot be gleaned from the scholarly literature. It would be irresponsible not to point out this important factor. First-person voices must be sought whenever possible. The emotional reactions that words convey cannot do justice to them, yet as an imperfect system of recording them, they bring us to the scene of the violence.

This chapter addresses a select number of topics due to limited space, but it does not take away from its importance. The two remaining chapters that follow offer recommendations that can be shaped to be included in this chapter, so readers interested in research must not despair. Research rests at the heart of any undertaking to make community changes; research on the death care sector, not unexpectedly, brings challenges and rewards.

Gun Violence Research as a Subfield of Various Disciplines

There is nothing about gun violence that precludes limiting who can be involved in stemming its immediate destruction and aftermath. This field's reach is only limited by our imagination and willingness to entertain new vistas. The following discussion on public memory and corresponding discourse broadens our vision of this field, with communities and society being beneficiaries.

Public memory can be viewed as manifestation of collective memory that can be applied to institutions, communities, and individuals (Phillips, 2004). I associate the act of destroying or erasing public memory with wars and enslavement (Araujo, 2020), as in this country. However, destroying or killing of the public memory of a deceased individual is a significant form of violence that needs to be recognized as such (Blatt, 2023). To think otherwise would classify this act as a misdemeanor and be a disservice to the individual being slandered, their families, and the neighborhood they called home.

Readers must not be surprised to think of cemetery studies as a subfield of historical archaeology (Veit, 2023). I am arguing, in this recommendation, for this field to expand its scope and include urban gun violence, usually attributed to gangs, as a subfield to categorize the emerging scholarship that will undoubtedly emerge in the next decade. Sociology and criminology, too, must think about this subfield due to its increasing prominence in urban areas of the country experiencing an expansion of gun deaths no longer limited to a distinct geographical space such as neighborhoods.

Bates (2024) discusses the challenges we face in listening to the voices of those who lost a loved one to violence, and in this case mothers, speaking to the experiences of countless individuals in the gun violence field and the challenges they face in living life after the loss of someone near:

> No matter how many times I have them, my interviews with mothers who have lost children to gun violence never get easier… The hardest part for me is feeling that I'm invading someone's grief, or leeching off it… Recently, I spoke with a mother whose son was killed

> in 2023 in New York City. He was 28 years old and lived most of his life in the Bronx. She said he wasn't a criminal but would hang out with the guys who were 'up to no good.' He was shot after an argument on a corner. I usually start these interviews by asking the mother about their son's childhood and a favorite memory, so things aren't too heavy initially. In this case, it didn't matter how I started the call. She cried the entire interview. I've talked with uncles and cousins who've lost multiple friends, seen people get shot or have been robbed at gunpoint themselves, and their responses were rather matter-of-fact. I think the reason is that although we've been around gun violence for years, we're fortunate that no one in our immediate family has been killed by gunfire.

We cannot work in this field from the confines of an office without needing to venture out into communities and talking to gun violence survivors either as primary or secondary victims. Those in the field cannot turn off our recorders at the end of the day and go back to routine tasks that await us. We, too, have our lives altered, reinforcing the importance of tapping voices that often go unheard by outsiders. Using adolescents as researchers is one example of pushing the envelope, but with much emotional support. Supporting youth-led research, for example, opens the door for the creation of a cadre of community-based researchers helping us gain insights into gun violence through the eyes and ears of youth (Marsh et al., 2024), symbolizing the key goals of community-centered programming. Uplifting youth voices represents a significant strategy regardless of the social problem or issue confronting them and their community (Checkoway, 2024).

Gun violence is too important to be limited to one profession or school of thought. The same can be said for research, as argued in this section. Further, it calls for both quantitative and qualitative approaches to help paint a picture of the challenges that we face in addressing prevention and the dire consequences it causes for families, communities, and the nation at large.

Capturing Narratives of Community Gun Violence

Stories have always captured my attention, and stories of community gun violence illustrate its far reaches. The broader the reach of capturing these stories, the more complete a picture we can obtain. Further, research must be undertaken with rather than for communities, and Ceccato and Westman (2024, p.14) stated this well: "Research is unanimous about the need to engage local stakeholders, such as community members, city leadership and the business community."

Gun violence narratives at final rites ceremonies must not be minimized or lost in the rush to craft interventions. This requires qualitative research uplifting these voices and stories to increase our understanding of how gun violence during this time period is different from gun violence in other settings and events. Capturing a longitudinal picture guides us in crafting interventions over a lifespan (Zimmerman et al., 2024).

A comprehensive understanding of community gun violence cannot be captured by what has happened in a day, week, month, or year, or from one vantage point in time, most likely the present. It necessitates taking a historical stance to grasp and appreciate how different layers of this violence have been stacked on over and over countless years and decades to fully understand how a community has suffered. It is never based on one incident, day, month, or year. It is a lifetime of trauma. True, we cannot go back in time and reverse the harm caused. We can, however, shape current efforts with a deep understanding and respect for the past.

The gun violence field must be assiduous in capturing the stories of victims of violence, as argued by Joshua Harris-Till, to be shared with current and future residents, normalizing these voices in the process (Everytown Research, 2021): "Some people describe the sound as a car backfiring. Others, popcorn on a hot fire. To me, though, gunshots were the soundtrack of my childhood … We don't have to grow like I did, with gunshots a more common refrain than ice cream truck songs on warm summer days … Our stories matter. We're not just dots on a map. And the continued, shared trauma of normalized gun violence in Black communities—it's a burden we shouldn't have to bear." That, readers, is community trauma!

A vision of "community" cannot be limited to formal institutions to be successful in stemming gun violence and helping victims at the local level. It is the equivalent of city government in communities experiencing numerous fires set by an arsonist; it cannot exclusively focus on individual fires and neglect to capture the arsonists setting the fires, for instance. Communities must be expected and supported to play an influential role in helping authorities address the causes of these fires. Stories help humanize earthly experiences and shape our interventions, allowing us to create a wider net of who should play a prominent role in addressing this public help challenge.

Research on Death Care Staff Burnout

Although burnout is a concept often applied in the helping professions, funeral and mortuary workers, too, suffer from this outcome due to stigma and incivility (Guidetti et al., 2021). Staff burnout in death care services has escaped scholarly attention in the United States, which caught me by surprise. I consulted the international literature to find research on this subject. This neglect includes what strategies have been attempted and succeeded in identifying and stemming these mental health consequences, particularly involving gun violence. In many ways, it is a "brave new world," and this raises the question as to why. Systematic data gathering and analysis on this phenomenon has not been done. Significant research funding is needed for testing interventions that take into account where they share similarities to those in the trauma field and where they present unique circumstances in the United States.

Further, it raises questions of what do we do about it? We may argue that this industry is profit-making, and it is incumbent on them to find solutions to the challenges they are facing, as in the case of any other business. However, although correct on the profit statement, death care, as previously argued, is not your ordinary "business," and I think most readers can agree with that stance. It certainly is not a high-paying profession to go along with a corresponding high level of prestige and privilege. What motivates those to seek a career in this sector remains generally unknown.

Exposure to death and bereavement does not necessarily turn out to be all negative. In fact, this exposure can be associated with "positive psychological development and personal growth" (Guidetti et al., 2021), lowering the anxiety of this life stage. It demystifies rituals associated with how deaths can be handled well from a socio-cultural standpoint. When this mourning process is mishandled or severely interrupted, as in the case of gun violence at a death ceremony, the opposite can occur.

Expanding how we conceptualize gun violence and corresponding deaths by taking into account new venues and contexts for it to transpire pushes the proverbial envelope in the field. Yes, there is always a high degree of anxiety accompanying any pushing of boundaries. However, there is no alternative other than to do so. Further, "gallows" humor can be found among cemetery, funeral, mortuary, and crematorium workers and others exposed to death, bereavement, and human suffering, providing insights into daily stresses they must contend with in performing their duties (Grandi et al., 2021). Similar humor can be found among those in high stress occupations because of how it helps mitigate tension inherent in their occupation.

Gallows humor is a coping strategy that we turn to in difficult moments or circumstances, allowing us to continue to function under very difficult circumstances (Lambert South et al., 2022, p.851): "In many cultures, death is a difficult or frightening topic to discuss with others … When communicating about difficult issues like death and dying, people may use several coping strategies to manage their discomfort. In particular, they may use humor, which provides a means for relieving emotions and fostering positive interactions with others."

Of course, there are other constructive and even reckless ways to "relieve" stress, such as engaging in sports or using mind-altering drugs. This dimension of the death care sector remains underresearched. Guidetti et al. (2021), in a rare study of funeral and mortuary workers and occupational burnout in Italy, found that stigma consciousness, supervisor incivility, and work-to-family negative spillover influenced levels of burnout. Gun violence was not part of their experiences, which brings a potentially deadly external factor. Those in the funeral field must contend with stigma and other occupational hazards that spill over into other arenas in their lives.

This book expands the gun violence field, singling out a variety of key institutions and professions, such as social work (Conrick et al., 2024; Sharpe, 2024), because of their unique community contributions, needs, and positions, including current community efforts to support them in carrying out their critical roles. Further, community institutions have started to purposefully get involved in sponsoring activities, bringing them into high-profile and prominent positions in addressing gun violence at the local level. This field can no longer wait patiently on the sidelines for the human services sector to knock on the door, undertake assessments, and initiate projects to help them navigate these stormy and dangerous seas.

Any change in thinking necessitates a tremendous amount of energy, time, and an expectation of institutional push back because challenging conventional thinking is rarely done without resistance. This conceptualization brings the death sector into a comprehensive system of care that is unconventional. Readers, regardless of practice and academic backgrounds, must rethink their views of the gun violence field (shift paradigms) and who should be at the table of decision-making. The person at the head of the table must represent the community, with the "supporting cast" expanded to include new sectors. New members can bring excitement, leading to bold initiatives. They can also lead to a learning cycle and an ability to overcome stereotypes. This balancing act is unavoidable but essential.

Being open to "new" and even "bold" approaches in unconventional arenas, including a willingness to accept and challenge conventional views, opens this practice field to innovative approaches, with all of the excitement and, unfortunately, trepidation that is to be expected. I say this being very cognizant of the challenges a "pushing the envelope" viewpoint brings. However, it is important to remember that I am not saying, "do this alone." Rather, there are countless like-minded individuals out there willing to take the least traveled path, so to speak. We must find them and join forces. I believe that the salience of this problem, by how it touches so many families, will cause residents and institutions to come forth and express willingness to collaborate on community projects, particularly when conceptualized by the community.

Conclusion

I hope that readers see the wisdom of why I wanted to highlight Jacksonville beyond seeking a broader geographical representation. Gun-related violence can take many forms beyond actual gunfire. A symbolic act intended to perpetrate psychological harm can lead to actual gun violence. Soiling a person's reputation is an act of violence because of how it harms their loved ones and their memory. Guns are part of the urban violence scene, permeating the air that we breathe. Social media, too, can be a weapon that causes massive destruction. In this case, soiling the reputation of a dead person and seeking to harm those who loved him, which in all likelihood is a young male victim.

We are at a point for paying attention to how we educate the field and the community to better address gun violence through research that will answer key questions from a community's standpoint. Educational recommendations, which follow in the next chapter, will cover a wide terrain, involving formal and informal efforts shaped by what communities want and need to carry out interventions that best meet local needs.

References

Araujo, A. L. (2020). *Slavery in the age of memory: Engaging the past*. Bloomsbury Publishing.

Bancalari, P., Sommer, M., & Rajan, S. (2022). Youth exposure to endemic community gun violence: A systematic review. *Adolescent Research Review, 7*(3), 383–417.

Bates, J. (2024, May 14). *Disrupting gun violence: A whole-community approach*. https://www.thirteen.org/blog-post/disrupt-gun-violence-community-approach/

Blatt, M. H. (2023). The second stage of violence: An excerpt from violence and public memory. *Parks Stewardship Forum, 39*(3).

Brandolino, A., deRoon-Cassini, T. A., Biesboer, E. A., Tomas, C. W., Woolfolk, M., Wakinekona, N. A., et al. (2024). Improved follow-up care for gun violence survivors in the Trauma Quality of Life Clinic. *Trauma Surgery & Acute Care Open, 9*(1), e001199.

Ceccato, V., & Westman, J. (2024). Where does firearm-related violence occur in cities? *Journal of Planning Literature, 08854122231219918.*

Checkoway, B. (2024). *Youth dialogues on race and ethnicity: Challenging segregation and strengthening diversity*. Oxford University Press.

Conrick, K. M., McCollum, O., Porter, S. F., St. Vil, C., Kanuha, V. K., Rowhani-Rahbar, A., & Moore, M. (2024). Preventing firearm injuries and deaths among clients: An action plan model for social workers. *Social Work, swae050.*

Dillard, D., Henderson, H., Mangum, M., Rice, J., II, & Goldstein, A. D. (2023). Unlocking gun-violence solutions: The necessity and power of lived experience. *American Journal of Qualitative Research, 7*(4), 182–202.

Everytown Research. (2021, May 27). *Invisible wounds: Gun violence and community trauma theory among Black Americans*. https://everytownresearch.org/report/invisible-woundsgun-violence-and-community-trauma-among-black-americans/

Grandi, A., Guidetti, G., Converso, D., Bosco, N., & Colombo, L. (2021). I nearly died laughing: Humor in funeral industry operators. *Current Psychology, 40*, 6098–6109.

Guidetti, G., Grandi, A., Converso, D., Bosco, N., Fantinelli, S., Zito, M., & Colombo, L. (2021). Funeral and mortuary operators: The role of stigma, incivility, work meaningfulness and work–family relation to explain occupational burnout. *International Journal of Environmental Research and Public Health, 18*(13), 6691.

Inklebarger, T. (2018, May 29). Gang burials a problem in western suburbs. County begins work in preparation of new funeral task force. *Forest Park Review*. https://www.forestparkreview.com/2018/05/29/gang-burials-a-problem-in-western-suburbs/

Lambert South, A., Elton, J., & Lietzenmayer, A. M. (2022). Communicating death with humor: Humor types and functions in death over dinner conversations. *Death Studies, 46*(4), 851–860.

Malone, N., Cannon, B., Wright, C. J., Peterson, R. L., Verty, V. P., Brown, J. K., et al. (2024). Mental health first aid for black populations: Recommendations from the neighborhood healers project. *The Counseling Psychologist, 00110000241252418.*

Marsh, L. T. S., Haynes, J. D., Belkin, L. D., & Scott, J. (2024). Confronting gun violence through youth-led participatory action research as a form of critical allyship with black youth: Insights for policymakers. The Congressional Black Caucus Foundation, Inc.(CBCF), 66.

Noorman, K., Davidson, K. M., Fridel, E. E., Arrigo, S., Strickland, R., Pesta, G. B., & Blomberg, T. G. (2025). Confronting community gun violence through research translation: A case study of challenges and facilitators. *American Journal of Criminal Justice*, 1–25.

Oppenheim, S., Webb, L., Testa, A., Fix, R. L., Clary, L., Mendelson, T., & Jackson, D. B. (2024). Police violence exposure and traumatic stress among youth: A systematic review. *Trauma, Violence, & Abuse, 15248380241255735.*

Phillips, K. R. (Ed.). (2004). *Framing public memory*. University of Alabama Press.

Sharpe, T. L. (2024). Building a legacy of research for black survivors of homicide victims: A call to action for social work. *Journal of the Society for Social Work and Research, 15*(3), 000–000.

Urbanik, M. M., & Roks, R. A. (2021). Making sense of murder: The reality versus the realness of gang homicides in two contexts. *Social Sciences, 10*(1), 17.

Veit, R. (2023). New perspectives in cemetery studies: A review essay. *International Journal of Historical Archaeology*, 1–12.

Zimmerman, G. M., Fridel, E. E., & Trovato, D. (2024). Disproportionate burden of violence: Explaining racial and ethnic disparities in potential years of life lost among homicide victims, suicide decedents, and homicide-suicide perpetrators. *PLoS One, 19*(2), e0297346.

Chapter 10
Education

Introduction

This chapter on education is not limited to the academic field, as also argued in the previous chapter on research (Chap. 9), although this arena plays an influential role in carrying out many of these recommendations. Innovative strategies and projects are destined to occur at the community level, with educational institutions playing collaborative roles (Staton et al., 2024) in advancing the gun violence field in the death care sector. I say this not because of my history as an academic. Rather, innovative projects ultimately fall within the realm of practitioners, with education playing a supportive role in preparing them for the road ahead, which is demanding and challenges us in ways that we never could even imagine.

DeReef (2023), for example, describes the potential contributions of trainings that can lead to theory development in the field as more research is devoted to the training and development of street outreach workers and curriculum to address urban community gun violence. Exchange of curriculum to allow localities to select the features that best meet local needs is very much in order. A similar model can be developed to bridge the gap between the death care sector and local street outreach models.

We must endeavor to broaden our vision of who is entrusted with dealing with the aftermath of gun violence ("*dirty work*"). The educational arena in addressing gun violence, for example, must be broad and extend beyond the "helping professions," such as master of public affairs programs, to better prepare governmental staff to address the emotional toll it takes for those practicing in urban areas with high gun violence, for example (Zavattaro et al., 2024). This chapter, nevertheless, focuses on the most obvious professions due to limited space.

© The Author(s), under exclusive license to Springer Nature Switzerland AG 2025

M. Delgado, *The Death Care Industry and Urban Gun Violence*,
https://doi.org/10.1007/978-3-031-95682-9_10

Foundation for Educational Recommendations

Preparing future practitioners and academics for the urban gun violence field is an immense responsibility for helping professions, and that is certainly the case with social work, for example (Hawley-Bernardez et al., 2024). This recommendation is immediate but with profound long-term ramifications, which should not be surprising. Again, starting with a respect for communities will stand as a cornerstone of any of these efforts. Having the community as an integral part of a team is an essential step in ensuring that the ultimate beneficiaries are at the table of decision-makers.

Readers may be surprised that there is such a field as "death practitioners and scholars," signifying a reservoir of knowledge that many of us are new to in this arena and a potential bridge between the gun violence field and the death care field. Reaching out to this field brings beneficial educational benefits to both sides of the equation of urban gun violence. Developing working relationships between these two worlds must be viewed developmentally through meetings, consultation, workshops, and even conferences. Building a foundation based on mutual trust and respect is essential in any endeavor and the proverbial "glue," it bears noting.

A great deal of attention has been paid to the African-American community in this book for very good reason. The Latino community, too, has suffered from gun violence, although without the benefit of receiving national attention in identifying their unique plight (American Progress, 2022):

> Although these high-profile shootings garnered significant public attention, the effect of gun violence on Hispanic communities is often left out of national conversations. Hispanic people, particularly Hispanic youth, are disproportionately affected by firearm violence in the United States. From 1999 to 2020, an estimated 74,522 Hispanic people in the United States died from gun violence, with violent homicides accounting for 60 percent of all gun deaths among Hispanic populations.[6] The latest available data suggest that these disparities are only growing: From 2014 to 2020, the number of Hispanic people who died due to gun violence rose by 66 percent, increasing at nearly twice the rate of gun deaths nationally.[7] In 2020, gun violence killed 5,003 Hispanic Americans, a record number that averages to 13 people per day.[8]

Gun violence within Latino neighborhoods brings challenges in meeting the needs of victims. Language and cultural barriers, not to mention documented status, all converge to make seeking justice and protection from law enforcement a challenge, to put it mildly. Cultural customs and values make last rites ceremonies challenging in neighborhoods where funeral homes owned and operated by Latinos are very rare. Where not available, they must rely on last-rite services being provided by those with little or no knowledge of their customs and traditions.

The question of whether children should be involved in viewing a corpse during a final-rites ceremony is one that anyone who has worked in the gun violence field has had to confront, particularly in the case of a parent or a sibling (Malachi, 2024) being buried. There is a recognition that bereavement and reactions to grief among children and adolescents are influenced by their developmental stage, bringing great challenges for the death care sector (Revet et al., 2020). Preparing the death care sector to help parents can be a multifaceted goal, involving members of the death care sector. The same can be said for siblings.

The recommendation to bring the death care sector and the human services sector closer together to improve final-rites events is not new. Rumbold et al. (2021), for example, advance the notion of building community partnerships between the death care sector and community organizations involved in end-of-life issues by redefining the role of this field to improve the functions of educating and facilitating service provision to the bereaved.

There is no disputing that the death of children brings an intense set of dynamics for the death care industry. Pediatric oncologists, for example, face particular challenges in carrying out their responsibilities. One study (Schoenbine et al., 2023) found that they will attend at least one of their patient's funerals, highlighting how children's deaths are special, much in similarity to the other professions touched upon in this book.

Those of us outside of the Black Church, for instance, may have a common perception that this institution has historically and currently been well positioned to help their membership with individual and communal grief related to the death of loved ones. Johnston (2024, p.34), nevertheless, cautions us to carefully question this perception, arguing that we must reconsider how individual and communal mourning is inadequate, making this holy institution need improvements to make it a refuge and healing center, noting:

> As pastors, we must acknowledge all of the different ways of recovery from the heart's difficulties. Whether as the closing of a funeral sermon or the closing of a regularly scheduled worship service, a ritual of lament will benefit as many people as possible if not more than the joyous opening praise service. Preaching that makes space for grief and the inclusion of grief rituals in African American worship services is a powerful tool for the African American preacher. It recognizes the humanity of those living in a society that believes them otherwise capable of suppressing the most normal of all human emotions.

I wonder whether the same can be said for Latino houses of worship, raising profound implications for service delivery. Latino churches outside of the Catholic realm are making significant inroads into this community (Delgado, 2025), and Latinos, too, have had to contend with gun violence in their communities. Those fleeing their home countries, for instance, may also be leaving behind gun violence and gangs.

There is acknowledgement that faith-based responses in the aftermath of gun violence must not stop at performing last rites, extending to helping those who have lost loved ones to this violence, making this sector an instrumental part of their recovery (Galiatsatos et al., 2021). Houses of worship are well positioned to help second victims obtain emotional support for those concerned about being labeled as "mentally ill." However, those providing these services need to be supported, too. Houses of worship, in essence, become mental health outposts and have been identified as partners in helping survivors made vulnerable to gun violence.

Memorials, sometimes referred to as "commemorative architectures" or "memorial architecture," can take many forms, as evidenced in Philadelphia and conceptualized as an educational tool to pay respect to those murdered by guns during the past calendar year and to spark discussion of how to stop urban gun violence (Heading God's Call, 2024): "**A Memorial to the Lost®** is a unique, visible education tool developed by Heeding to honor victims of gun violence and their surviving families. T-shirts with names and dates of those murdered by gun violence during a previous year in a designated area are displayed in front of a congregation's building or in a public space where community members can experience in a tangible way the loss of life and disruption of lives that gun violence creates. Often, people will stop their car after driving by and return to see exactly what's being portrayed; they will walk among the shirts, pause and pray, sometimes even finding the name of a loved one or neighbor. The Philadelphia Memorial usually contains close to 300 names reminding us of the immensity of the problem." Memorials often take on significant local influences, and we must eschew viewing these sites from a cookie-cutter approach. Nevertheless, they share many similar goals.

Sponsoring Educational Workshops for the Death Care Sector

Expanding where education transpires is essential in moving the gun violence field forward as is evident by the spotlight put on various forms of education in this chapter. Having educational workshops at various levels and settings is important because gun violence and the death care sector are not relegated to one segment of society, increasing the likelihood that all who need this information are able to get it. Further, this means that this education must be offered in community settings and in non-stigmatizing ways to reach a broad sector of the field and community.

These workshops can transpire in settings that are geographically, operationally, culturally, and psychologically (stigma-free) accessible. Public libraries, for example, come to mind as possible sites for these trainings. These sites generally are well situated within urban communities, are politically non-aligned with any community faction, have space for workshops, and are non-stigmatizing to be seen at. Libraries, of course, are not the only sites for these trainings. Readers have a general sense of sites conducive to community workshops.

Funeral parlors, not surprisingly, also bring many of these same qualities, for example, and further destigmatize these settings, helping to break down potential attitudinal barriers to engagement. Needless to say, education can transpire in various forms and settings not normally associated with this activity.

Training/Consultation on Community Trauma

Training can be conceptualized as a form of education as well as an intervention. Introducing this topic as an intervention highlights the importance of thinking about this activity of bringing about organizational/community changes. I wonder out loud how well personnel in the death care sector are familiar with mental health services; conversely, we can also ask what trauma staff know about what staff involved in death services encounter and their needs. Self-care is clearly a subject with great applicability to this sector, as it is in the formal care arena. There is no denying that these two worlds coexist, dealing with the same victims, community, and circumstances.

Provision of training and consultation is a relatively inexpensive form of service delivery. I have often used these approaches as a means of putting my "foot in the door," so to speak, and establishing assessments and eventual service delivery requiring a more extensive commitment of time and effort. Any process that allows an assessment of merit for an extensive and more labor-intensive working relationship without making a long-term commitment benefits all parties involved.

In-service training in the trauma sector, for example, would benefit from having personnel from the death services sector present, as well as having staff from trauma services do in-service training in the death sector. I have always found that doing trainings is an excellent way of breaking down barriers and stereotypes one sector may have about the other, facilitating relationship-building based on mutual trust. These trainings do not have to be labor-intensive either. However, when training groups are well conceived, it not only increases competencies in the field, but also breaks down stereotypes that interfere with establishing collaborations.

Bocanegra and Aguilar (2024) address the importance of the relationship between those in the community violence field and those they serve, identifying four key interrelated themes with significant bearing on those embracing this form of practice and the stressors they can expect to encounter in carrying out their roles: (1) "work as mission"; (2) "tethered healing ('a mutually reinforcing healing dynamic that evolves in their relationship');" (3) "tethered harm" (relapsing back to street life); and (4) "falling back" (potentially experiencing harm and even death). Work as a mission will not come as any great surprise to anyone devoting their life to work that is under-recognized by society. Those in the death care sector experience these stressors, too.

The voices of those left behind to pick up the pieces of gun violence often go unheard and are generally left to their own devices to sound the alarm of the devastation and trauma it has caused families (Lund et al., 2024). Community trauma, as discussed earlier, is an immensely powerful construct when discussing gun violence regardless of where it transpires, but it takes on added significance in urban centers. The immensity of its power is only matched by the challenges it presents to the academy and practice field in understanding its influence and how best to address it when discussing gun violence (Foiles, 2019).

Community trauma is worthy of research funding and projects testing new approaches to helping communities heal from gun violence. Community trauma requires the same level of funding as other forms of trauma. The vastness that community trauma encompasses necessitates long-term funding rather than funding limited to several years, which is customary. Further, community trauma requires a multidisciplinary approach that enlists community members as part of the research team, helping ensure that the many nuances associated with this trauma get captured.

Trauma centers need to play a pivotal or coordinating role in these research undertakings, particularly Level I and II centers when providing 24/7 emergency response services. However, there is no denying that these centers are currently underfunded, making it difficult to expand their mission to include community trauma (Fracasso & Ahmed, 2024): "Costs associated with trauma center operation have risen over the past few years in association with growing patient volumes and inflation. Documentation regarding costs for trauma center operations is sparse, and there exists a large variance between reported numbers based on their region. In most cases, the greatest proportion of funds are spent on clinical personnel while the smallest fraction is dedicated to educational and prevention programs. Studies confirm that as a product of these rising costs and a lack of state and federal funding that trauma centers remain uniquely financially vulnerable."

Further challenging us in understanding community trauma is the importance of a multidisciplinary approach that captures the historical nuances of gun violence in urban communities of color. This challenge necessitates making urban historians part of these efforts, in addition to other professions normally not found around the table in discussions of community trauma. Urban gun violence is too important a public health problem to limit who is "authorized" to research trauma.

Death Care Sector "STOP THE BLEED" Campaign

This is a good point to uplift a case illustration of an intervention that has appeal across geographical settings but with particular relevance for urban settings. Bleeding and gun violence go hand in hand. Thus, the nature of gun violence necessitates that victims have immediate access to medical treatment to increase the likelihood of surviving at the scene of the shooting until they can obtain medical treatment. Successful intervention at a gun shooting represents the essence of any early intervention campaign (Delgado, 2022, p.137): "Blood is symbolic of life, and any campaign to save human life embracing blood as a key element brings saliency and symbolism to gun violence campaigns."

The Stop the Bleed campaign is a community educational intervention that is over 10 years old, and this is a testament to its success, gaining currency across the nation (Rossaint et al., 2013): (1) increase knowledge, self-efficacy, and willingness of individuals living in communities most impacted by gun violence to perform bystander bleeding control and (2) build trust and familiarity between the community and first responders. This campaign is best implemented when sponsored by well-known and respected community institutions, breaking down potential obstacles based on suspicions of outside organizations.

The Stop the Bleed campaign is international in origin with a goal of reducing the number of patients who die within 24 h of arriving at a medical facility, taking center stage in this country because of gun violence. This goal necessitates that an intervention occur immediately at the scene until an ambulance can arrive. The effectiveness of Stop the Bleed campaigns is enhanced when they are locally based and sponsored by well-respected local organizations. Nothing about a community without the community!

Quick medical care access upon a gun injury is greatly influenced by geospatial access to care, as in the case of Philadelphia (Byrne et al., 2022) and other high gun violence cities across the nation. It is important to note that cemeteries, for example, are not easily accessible to ambulance services, making intervention that much more important when compared to a house of worship or funeral home, which, in all likelihood, are more easily geographically accessible to hospitals.

There are two primary goals of Stop the Bleed programs, which can be classified as a community engagement model (Williams et al., 2024): "(1) increase knowledge, self-efficacy, and willingness of individuals living in communities most impacted by gun violence to perform bystander bleeding control; and (2) build trust and familiarity between the community and first responders."

More specifically, Stop the Bleed is a graphic description of what this intervention's goal is, with campaigns embracing three particular skills (Jacobs et al., 2022): "First and foremost, the Stop the Bleed® training course teaches immediate responders how to recognize life-threatening hemorrhage and how to control bleeding in an injured patient. Three main skills are emphasized including application of direct pressure, wound packing, and the use of a tourniquet." These are specific knowledge and skill sets that broaden a community's competencies in this life-and-death arena.

This program has been tailored to specific systems such as schools, for example. However, I am calling for a campaign specifically focused on the death care sector in communities with high rates of gun violence. Villegas et al. (2020) address this campaign's success on hemorrhage cessation, but there is still room for improvement by expanding the terrain to the death care sector and the uniqueness of these settings.

Readers interested in developing a more nuanced understanding and insights into the world of those practitioners in the death sector are encouraged to read Campbell's (2023) book *All the Living and the Dead: An Exploration of the People Who Make Death Their Life's Work*. This sector, although focusing on a limited arena in my book, consists of many other areas, such as mass fatality investigators, embalmers, and executioners, for example. The author seeks to answer a key question: why would anyone choose to make a living doing this work? There certainly is a call for similar books on people of color in this sector. Understanding these motivations helps the gun violence field better meet its specific needs and recruit a workforce for this field, which only promises to increase due to demographic trends increasing the number of people of color and urbanization.

Self-Help Organizations

Readers are familiar with various forms of self-help organizations, which are a locally based intervention. These organizations have a long history in our society devoted to a variety of major problems. Self-help organizations are generally found in urban centers of the country, with various manifestations and names (Borkman et al., 2020). These organizations also reach survivors of gun violence, their families, and, from help-seeking perspectives, can be the first efforts to secure aid (Delgado, 2022). They have emerged to meet unmet needs in what are often formal resource-poor communities.

I am a big advocate of self-help organizations because they serve as a valuable bridge between the formal world of service providers and communities, assuming roles as educators and social brokers. I like to say that we need to identify them, support them, and use them whenever possible to help ensure that we are grounded. They are best thought of as indigenous community assets that have emerged to reach those who fall between the cracks at a moment of great need.

Parents grieving children lost to gun violence, for example, are not monolithic in how they mourn, opening the door for each family to bring their distinctive approach to mourning. The story of Johnny Johnson (killed in 2017) touches upon many of the themes raised in this chapter and throughout this book (Colombini, 2023): "Johnny Johnson is wearing a T-shirt with a smiling teenage boy's face on it. That same face is etched on a tombstone a few feet away, framed by a pair of basketball hoops. Johnson's son, Jayquon, died on New Year's Day nearly seven years ago. He was 17. Jayquon, known as 'Quon,' was a high school sophomore and rising basketball star. Another teen shot him in a Tampa-area suburb during an argument over drugs. 'My life was never the same since that phone call,' said Johnson, speaking from the cemetery where his son is buried. 'Even though plenty of my peers' kids was murdered and gunned down and stuff, so it wasn't new to me, but there's a difference when it knocks on your door.'" Johnny Johnson illustrates this observation by wearing a T-shirt showing a smiling teenage boy's face on it, similar to that etched on his tombstone, which is framed by a pair of basketball hoops.

Parents involved in self-help organizations such as "Rise to Peace," based in Tampa, Florida, capture how these efforts seek to fill a vacuum in helping loved ones navigate the trials and tribulations of life without a child, as noted by Johnny Johnson (Colombini, 2023): "We've been sentenced to life without our loved ones, just like them, so that makes us always available, 365 days a year, 24 hours a day." This commitment is best made by parents and other loved ones still on the journey of recovery. Helping others in this journey aids them in the healing journey, too. It is easy to see how an entire community can benefit as a result.

O'Neill et al. (2020) point out that gun violence survivors attempting to recover from that experience will do so back in the community where they likely experienced this violence, but also in all likelihood home of happy memories, too. Recovery in a "neutral" or even a "therapeutic" space is not possible for all but only a few who are lucky to do so. These individuals can be assets in a fight against gun violence if they receive the needed help that is required. Those who were shot at a death sector ceremony, in turn, are uniquely qualified to help staff mount initiatives with this segment as a focus, bringing experiential expertise to the table. This unique experience separates them from countless other victims but in different settings. They can more effectively act as a bridge for others who distrust the medical/mental health field, for instance.

Philadelphia, Pennsylvania's Mothers in Charge is one of numerous examples across the nation of how gun murders of children can be a key motivator for bringing together mothers in support of each other to share a common bond and engage in activities to reduce gun violence in their neighborhoods (Adams & Marin, 2024). Sadly, a comparable gathering for fathers and siblings could not be located, which doesn't mean that they do not exist. I simply could not find one. Although there is certainly a great need for this type of group because they can be, and have been, easily overlooked (Delgado, 2024; Panchal, 2024).

Although mothers' groups give the impression that only mothers are limited to this group, fathers and siblings, too, can join in many local instances. However, mothers are often in charge and thus well positioned to broker collaborations between the formal care sector and the death care sector. Tapping their experience, knowledge, and commitment makes them natural brokers. A point on self-help is in order. Sadly, self-help organizations, too, are not exempt from experiencing gun violence. That, on the surface, should not be surprising if last rites and the institutions performing them, too, are not exempt! The immensity of their mission matches the dangers they face. Self-help organizations, where they exist, must have a prominent place at the table of any intervention.

Urban Memorials as Educational Projects

Urban memorials can be conceptualized along a variety of perspectives. These memorials, however, have a place within an educational sphere. Commemorating the death of a loved one is an attempt to keep a memory alive to be shared with others, almost as if they are still among the living. We are very familiar with memorials of all kinds, and they are as old as the nation itself (Dory et al., 2003). They, of course, can have various manifestations. Memorials dedicated to loved ones can take many different forms and shapes, often reflecting cultural traditions and local urban contexts. They can take the form of money donated to establish a scholarship fund to support students, for example. Of course, these funds can also support lectureships and endowed university chairs by well-resourced donors. However, in low-resourced communities of color, they take the form of a physical alteration of the environment.

In urban communities, memorials generally take on a physical presence to remind us of a life lost and sorely missed. The nature of these memorials, in turn, can have various manifestations—from the painting of murals and establishing community gardens to honor those lost to gun violence, to exhibitions at local museums, schools, and houses of worship, for example. Some memorials are temporary, while others take on a more permanent status, depending upon financial resources and the significance of the person being memorialized. Further, they can take many different manifestations. Memorials can become a vehicle for enhancing local history, grounding past events within a context that helps unite generations.

The emergence of what are called "Object Collection Events" on gun violence, which are sometimes referred to as "symbolic cemeteries," is another art form, as discussed earlier regarding Boston, which addresses the pain this violence creates and the importance of safe spaces for these exhibitions (Dell'Aria, 2020). These collection events can be permanent and added to on a yearly basis or can ascend to become a traveling exhibit to multiple cities, allowing local sites to add to the exhibit.

Royster (2021) described the Dolls4Peace Memorial, another form of art project: "Areas that have historically struggled through racial segregation, poverty and disinvestment are most impacted by gun violence. The Dolls4Peace art action and memorial highlights the need for routine community-based art therapy in schools and communities to address trauma caused by gun violence. This community-based art making and sharing is needed not only for the youth, but also for families and teachers who are left to mend and pick up the pieces."

These spaces are meant to honor the deceased, allowing loved ones to expand awareness of these victims, and can be undertaken in a variety of places and spaces. However, they stand as testament to lives lost to families, loved ones, and their respective communities. Mind you, they are not meant to glorify but to honor, and there is a distinct difference between the two. Glorifying increases the likelihood of engendering further violence; honoring will have a less likelihood of causing further violence. Local circumstances, of course, will dictate whether this recommendation is feasible. Nevertheless, lives lost cannot be relegated to history. These memorials serve to remind communities of times that no one wishes to return to.

Memorials can be planned by a family and/or a community, in cases of a widely admired member, and anticipated to be part of the landscape in the case of cemeteries, taking various shapes (Goodnow, 2021, p. 1815): "Memorials in cemeteries function epideictically to commemorate the life and final resting place of the dead. In addition, permanent public memorials are often built at sites of national tragedy. These memorials are built on what is considered 'sacred ground.'"

These memorials can be spontaneous, too, and viewed through a variety of prisms, one of which is as sacred spaces for remembering the dead, often as a result of an unexpected violent act (Grider, 2022). Memorials, planned or unplanned, because of their symbolism, can be subject to vandalism as a means of furthering a public dispute and insulting the family of the deceased, in a similar fashion to what is happening concerning the vandalism of gravestones.

Gravestones often contain messages that symbolize who misses them and why, in addition to their names and dates of birth and death. These stones have been personalized to the deceased. Sadly, once again, memorials can be sites of further gun violence, as in the case of a Syracuse woman paying her respects for a fallen member of the community (Rubinstein et al., 2018). This shooting at an urban memorial can easily fall within the category of the other last rites sacred sites covered in this book.

Over 20 years ago (Delgado, 2003), I wrote a book titled *Death at an Early Age and the Urban Scene: The Case for Memorial Murals and Community Healing*. That book sought to capture the epidemic of drug overdoses and gun violence that dramatically altered what it meant to live in many of this nation's urban centers, such as Chicago, Illinois; Los Angeles, California; and New York, New York, and the need for families and other loved ones to keep their memories alive and help communities heal. However, gun violence at cemeteries, funeral homes, and houses of worship was not taking place, which is an indicator of how recent these shootings have emerged, reflecting on a dramatic shift as to what constitutes sacred ground and off-limits to this violence.

Visiting a cemetery was difficult (far away) and expensive where I was growing up, in addition to the importance of having them continue to have a presence where they were known and loved. Murals are a form of artwork, often with deep historical significance, and are sponsored or undertaken by families of the deceased. The location brings significant meaning to the deceased, such as on the side of a house where they lived, or even where they met their final moments on earth, for example.

Hunter (2022, p. 246) discusses the African-American Church as an Afrocentric sacred space and what makes it so and why it is an important aspect related to gun violence because of its centrality in countless lives: "A sacred space is a place created by a person (or people) who conducts an action important to him or her, practices a ritual, or simply makes a place where he or she can feel safe. To its user, this space is created, claimed, owned, and is made special compared to any other space or place. This space can be naturally created or physically constructed but will have substance and meaning for its users." Houses of worship can take their place alongside funeral homes and cemeteries as sacred places. Within the Black-American community, they ascend to even greater significance because of the paucity of institutions that they control and are integrally tied to their lives.

Black churches were originally constructed and financed by the enslaved and/or newly freed, making these places and structures as one of the few spaces owned, patronized, and operated by the Black community. This institutional foundation has largely remained to the present. However, it has faced numerous challenges over the past several centuries, including struggles for their very survival, resulting in their closures. Gun violence adds a new chapter in their struggles for literal and figurative survival in this society.

As already noted, it is impossible to separate Black-American funeral home history from this community's history of enslavement and segregation. The Black Church, too, faced similar challenges as newly emancipated Black Americans were forced to develop their own worship houses because of racial discrimination. Funeral homes and cemeteries, in turn, take on the added significance of being viewed as sanctuaries, much in similarity to houses of worship.

These spaces are not supposed to be attacked and be crime scenes; these spaces are best viewed as sacred spaces. Sanctuary spaces are rare in high-violence communities, so when they are attacked, it adds immensely to the misery index. This harm is not only immediate, but has immense long-range consequences. Urban communities without sanctuary spaces effectively resemble war scenes, compromising health and well-being for current and future generations. War results in the absence of safe spaces and a world devoid of love. In high-violence communities, the physical environment often takes on this semblance. Urban memorials, in a similar fashion to their better-known war memorials, can take various shapes. However, regardless of manifestations, they serve the same goals of making sure we do not forget.

Law Enforcement Role: "Can't Live with Them and Can't Live Without Them!"

Let's face it. It would be impossible to author this book without paying due attention to law enforcement. Development of successful collaborative projects will necessitate having local law enforcement to be partners in educational projects that will break down suspicion between communities and local police. The subject of law enforcement has been touched upon in various parts of this book but without the spotlight being put on them. Numerous books have been written about law enforcement at the local level for very good reasons. They are the face of government and how gun violence or not prioritized as a major problem in our society.

Further, and extremely important, we must not overlook a history of police distrust by the community (Andrade et al., 2021, p.260): "Effective community solutions require collaboration ... Problematically, the criminal justice and medical institutions, given their institutionalized racism and history of mistreatment of communities of color, suffer from distrust by the communities that they are attempting to serve..." The weight of this legacy cannot simply be put aside because we do not seek to perpetrate this injustice!

Some readers may view this recommendation with suspicion. Law enforcement can and must play a critical role in preventing gun violence at a last rites event. A police presence at a memorial service can prevent further gun violence, as in the case of Pennsylvania (Southard, 2024). Two teenagers were apprehended and a gun recovered by the police at a burial for a 13-year-old who had been shot and killed. However, police presence can also take on the semblance of a police state, taking away from a solemn occasion. Having educational projects as a precursor to joint projects can help break down stereotypes that hinder communication and trust, essential in any successful effort to stem gun violence at death care sites.

Expanding Views and Sites for Death Rituals

Death rituals exist for very good reason—they meet the needs of those left behind. These rituals are not relegated to particular sites, although there are places where they have a natural setting for them to take place. Death rituals are not restricted to death care settings and the ever-expansive nature of saying final goodbyes, necessitating grounding these acts within a broad scope to fully comprehend the multifaceted influence of gun violence (Jarrett, 2015):

> Pamela Rayner, one of the owners of the funeral home, remembers one mother who would not speak for 15 minutes when she came to arrange services for her son. At the funeral, she stood outside for 25 minutes before entering. 'It kind of got to me because I'm thinking to myself this is her only child,' Rayner said. 'Can you imagine not today, not tomorrow, but next week when everybody is gone and everybody is back to their old daily work, she has to go into their son's house, in their son's room, and start putting away his clothes.' She has seen mothers and grandmothers who have taken out life insurance on their own kids. She had to stop one funeral because of the threat of gang retaliation, and tell the mourners that for their own protection the service couldn't go on.

The heartbreak of a mother, or any other close relative, of losing a child cannot easily be put into words, regardless of a writer's ability. There is such a profound sense of sorrow that it is impossible to capture and put on paper. Words are not enough. The facial expressions and the difficulty of finding the "right" words that do justice to these feelings are impossible.

Funeral financial costs can be excessive, bringing up memories for me of having neighbors solicit funds by going door-to-door in my building asking for donations to bury a loved one. It is also not unusual to have family members of the deceased selling shirts and pins with the pictures or names of the deceased at services or at local establishments to help defray the costs of a funeral, as discussed earlier in this book. Fundraising comes in many different forms, accounting for local circumstances. Obviously, these actions go far beyond soliciting funds but also garnering emotional support in the process, which is arguably more important over the long run for loved ones.

This chapter and section have provided a broad sample of the types of education initiatives that are needed in fighting urban gun violence. Readers can no doubt see the blurring of lines between education and interventions, and that is to be expected. Reader imagination and creativity are essential in helping to increase the likelihood that educational undertakings will be successful in helping survivors and preventing further violence. The next and final chapter will focus squarely on what are "typical" forms of interventions.

Destigmatizing Funeral Homes: Field Trips?

Visiting a funeral home is never a go-to subject, and this hesitancy cannot be overlooked in this recommendation. I have always loved field trips throughout my entire formal education. I found them to break the routine of education, being exposed to new vistas, and a "fun" activity. Maybe some readers share this enthusiasm. How about taking a field trip to a local funeral parlor? Although funeral homes are integral to all communities and address universal needs, there is a phobia or stigma to how they are viewed that has isolated many of them from the social fabric of a neighborhood. Breaking down these negative perceptions is critical to achieving many of the recommendations outlined in this book. There has, nevertheless, been recognition of this situation in some communities.

Community organizations in high gun violence cities, for example, have started to sponsor field trips to funeral homes where youth are exposed to a lecture on gun violence, for example, educating them on the less "romanticized" and "glamorous" aspects of gun violence portrayed in television shows and movies, for example (McCray, 2023):

> Raise your hand if you know someone under the age of 21 who lost their life to violence," said Spoken Word artist Muhibb Dyer. The kids sat, and would eventually walk in front of, an open casket with a mirror inside, symbolizing what could happen if violence were to strike. 'It may be triggering for some people and if you need to walk out that's okay,' said one leader with EOP. The kids also heard from beloved Milwaukee Pastor Lovelace Redmond. 'It's going to take more than just the ministers, and the pastors in town, it's going to take things like this to happen,' said Pastor Redmond. Pastor Redmond has presided over Milwaukee funerals for decades.
>
> Pastor Redmond went on to note that over the past several years: "more mothers and fathers are burying their children. 'It is a problem, it's a big problem, because we are losing more young people now than ever before.' The service hitting close to some like 16-year-old Amere Watson. 'I know what it feels like to lose someone to violence.' Watson recently lost her mother due to domestic violence. She said she hopes her peers take Wednesday's message to heart. 'I just want them to know, like it's all fun and games until you're in a situation where you're losing your life., it's all heheh's and haha's and laughter until your friends are in that situation or you're face-to-face with death.'

The effectiveness of funeral homes' ventures remains to be measured by research. However, there is no denying that there is a high-violence community's willingness to try measures that fall out of the ordinary because they are facing extraordinary events and challenges, with no segment of the community having the luxury of sitting by the sidelines.

These and other types of "talks" are increasing in frequency and substance to help youth realize the consequences of gun violence are not to be romanticized. There is no glory in dying in a gun battle, with family and friends left behind to literally and figuratively pick up the pieces afterward and destined to have shrines dedicated to them in their homes. Youth exposure (level and type) to community violence is under-researched as a topic, let alone when it occurs at a sacred site (Bancalari et al., 2022). Visiting a funeral home and engaging with staff is one method to have youth and others understand that there is nothing romantic about death due to guns!

Community Workshops and Conferences

I debated whether to put this recommendation in the chapter on education or practice because it straddles both categories. I elected to go with the education chapter. Education is an intervention! How well it is carried out determines its impact on gun violence. It is also an intervention that can be relatively inexpensive with a prodigious potential outcome if well conceptualized and implemented. It allows potential participants to weigh whether or not the investment of time, which may be relatively short and time-limited, may lead to greater cooperation and commitment down the road.

I am sure most, if not all, readers have attended numerous conferences and workshops at the national, state, and local levels. Educational events provide opportunities to enhance knowledge and skills but also serve as a networking mechanism, allowing us to connect with other likeminded individuals that can be tapped when we return home to our own institutions. Most of these educational opportunities can be accessed through in person and via teleconference mechanisms. These connections ascend to greater importance than the newfound knowledge obtained.

Sponsoring community workshops and conferences that encourage participation from various sectors is a non-threatening way to break down stereotypes, helping establish connections between the death care sector, community-based organizations and concerned residents. There will be institutions within the death care sector that will show an interest in collaborating; others may take a wait-and-see attitude. Thus, starting with those businesses and institutions showing the greatest willingness to work together is the best way to start, and if successful, building upon these successes to reach out to others. The sponsors of these educational opportunities must be well respected within the community, bringing institutional legitimacy, which can vary according to local circumstances.

Bamwine et al. (2024) spotlight bereavement processes that Black-American adolescent male co-victims of a gun murder experience, identifying four themes that appear in this group and are worthy of being highlighted here: "(1) self-preservation through isolation, (2) finding sanctuary through shared narratives of loss, (3) freedom from the mind, and (4) post-traumatic growth (i.e., motivation, healing, resilience)." These themes will reappear in various forms in the final chapter on recommendations shaping practice for well-deserved reasons.

Conclusion

There is no denying the power of education, particularly when serving as a bridge between research and practice. Clearly, as evidenced in this chapter, education covers a very wide terrain, allowing for local circumstances to dictate the scope and nature of projects that can be initiated to expand the field of gun violence interventions. I am sure that some readers would have placed some of the categories covered in this chapter in other chapters. That is indicative of how flexible education can be viewed. The following final chapter, too, will further expand the field by introducing projects that allow for a wide variety of projects to unfold to meet community needs.

References

Adams, D., & Marin, M. (2024, April 15). Philadelphia gun violence victims find support through residents and nonprofits. *Wisconsin Public Radio*. https://www.wpr.org/news/philadelphia-gun-violence-victims-find-support-through-residents-and-nonprofits

American Progress. (2022, November 1). *Gun violence has a devastating impact on hispanic communities*. https://www.americanprogress.org/article/gun-violence-has-a-devastating-impact-on-hispanic-communities/

Andrade, E. G., Hayes, J. M., Wood, I., & Punch, L. J. (2021). Reducing the incidence and impact of gun violence through community engagement. In M. Crandall, S. Bonne, J. Bronson, & W. Kessel (Eds.), *Why we are losing the war on gun violence in the United States* (pp. 255–264). Springer.

Borkman, T., Munn-Giddings, C., & Boyce, M. (2020). Self-help/mutual aid groups and peer support: A literature review. *Voluntaristics Review, 5*(2–3), 1–219.

Byrne, J. P., Kaufman, E., Scantling, D., Tam, V., Martin, N., Raza, S., et al. (2022). Association between geospatial access to care and firearm injury mortality in Philadelphia. *JAMA Surgery, 157*(10), 942–949.

Colombini, S. (2023, December 13). Some families who lost their kids to gun violence channel their pain into action. *Health News Florida*. https://health.wusf.usf.edu/health-news-florida/2023-12-13/some-families-who-lost-their-kids-to-gun-violence-channel-their-pain-into-action

DeReef, V. P. (2023). *Standardizing the training of Chicago's street outreach community through the Metropolitan Peace Academy: A community of practice* (Doctoral dissertation, Adler University, Chicago, IL).

Delgado, M. (2022). *The silent epidemic of gun injuries: Challenges and opportunities for treating and preventing gun injuries*. Oxford University Press.

Delgado, M. (2024). *Urban public spaces, events, and gun violence: Block parties, funerals, mother's day, and other community events*. Springer Publishers.

Delgado, M. (2025). *When the Lord's House closes: Church closings and urban community practice*. Oxford University Press.

Dell'Aria, A. (2020). Loaded objects: Addressing gun violence through art in the gallery and beyond. *Palgrave Communications, 6*(1), 1–11.

Dory, K., Ruggiero, M., & Lavender, C. (2003). The history of memorials. *History, 401*, 9443.

Foiles, J. (2019). *This city is killing me: Community trauma and toxic stress in urban America*. Arcadia Publishing.

Fracasso, J. L., & Ahmed, N. (2024). Trauma centers: An underfunded but essential asset to the community. *Trauma Surgery & Acute Care Open, 9*(1), e001436.

Galiatsatos, P., Cudjoe, T. K., Bratcher, J., Heikkinen, P., Leaf, P., & Golden, S. H. (2021). Second victims: Aftermath of gun violence and faith-based responses. *Journal of Religion and Health, 60*, 1832–1838.

Goodnow, T. (2021). The silent witness project as rhetorical hybrid: Toward a theory of collective mourning. *American Behavioral Scientist, 65*(13), 1805–1819.

Hawley-Bernardez, A., Patton, J., Meza, C., & Gibbons, G. (2024). Addressing gun violence through social work education. *Social Work Education*, 1–14.

Heading God's Call. (2024). *Memorials to the lost. A public witness to gun violence*. Philadelphia Yearly Meeting of the Religious Society of Friends. https://www.pym.org/friends-ending-gun-violence/memorial-to-the-lost/

Hunter, C. (2022). The African American church house: A phenomenological inquiry of an Afrocentric sacred space. *Religions, 13*(3), 246.

Jacobs, L., Keating, J. J., Hunt, R. C., Butler, F. K., Pons, P. T., Gestring, M., et al. (2022). Stop the Bleed®. *Current Problems in Surgery, 59*(10), 101193.

Johnston, C. D. (2024). Grave preaching: Homiletical violence in the face of grief. *Theology Today, 81*(1), 27–34.

Malachi, A. N. (2024). *"The Forgotten Ones": Understanding the lived experience of losing a sibling to homicide through sense of community and mindfulness* (Doctoral dissertation, Point Park University, Pittsburgh, PA).

O'Neill, K. M., Vega, C., Saint-Hilaire, S., Jahad, L., Violano, P., Rosenthal, M. S., et al. (2020). Survivors of gun violence and the experience of recovery. *Journal of Trauma and Acute Care Surgery, 89*(1), 29–35.

Panchal, N. (2024). *The impact of gun violence on children and adolescents. The independent source for health policy research, polling, and news*. https://www.kff.org/mental-health/issue-brief/the-impact-of-gun-violence-on-children-and-adolescents/

Revet, A., Bui, E., Benvegnu, G., Suc, A., Mesquida, L., & Raynaud, J. P. (2020). Bereavement and reactions of grief among children and adolescents: Present data and perspectives. *L'encephale, 46*(5), 356–363.

Rossaint, R., Bouillon, B., Cerny, V., Coats, T. J., Duranteau, J., Fernández-Mondéjar, E., et al. (2013). The STOP the bleeding campaign. *Critical Care, 17*, 1–4.

Royster, R. (2021, April). Dolls4Peace memorial: Liberatory community art action and praxis. *Voices: A World Forum for Music Therapy, 21*(1).

Rubinstein, R. A., Lane, S. D., Mojeed, L., Sanchez, S., Catania, E., Jennings-Bey, T., et al. (2018). Blood in the rust belt: Mourning and memorialization in the context of community violence. *Current Anthropology, 59*(4), 439–454.

Rumbold, B., Lowe, J., & Aoun, S. M. (2021). The evolving landscape: Funerals, cemeteries, memorialization, and bereavement support. *OMEGA-Journal of Death and Dying, 84*(2), 596–616.

Schoening, D., Gerhart, J., McLean, K. A., deBettencourt, J., Dadrass, F., Molina, E., et al. (2023). Attending patient funerals as a follow-up practice of pediatric oncologists. *Illness, Crisis & Loss, 31*(1), 168–174.

Southard, A. (2024, August 23). 2 juveniles detained, gun found near funeral service for 13-year-old shooting victim. *(Local 21 News.com)*. https://local21news.com/news/local/2-juveniles-detained-gun-found-near-funeral-service-for-13-year-old-shooting-victim-steelton-teen-progress-avenue-gun-violence-naryah-wright-memorial-zion-church-police-investigating-susquehanna-township-pa.

Staton, A. R., Gilligan, T., & Kielty, M. (2024). Interprofessional and community collaboration in gun violence prevention and intervention. In J. Herron, S. R. Sartin, & S. R. (Eds.), *Impact of gun violence in school systems* (pp. 155–176). IGI Global.

Villegas, C. V., Gupta, A., Liu, S., Curren, J., Rosenberg, J., Barie, P. S., et al. (2020). Stop the bleed: Effective training in need of improvement. *Journal of Surgical Research, 255*, 627–631.

Williams, A., Evans, C., Nehra, D., Stadeli, K. M., Bulger, E. M., & Dicker, R. (2024). Building community: Community engagement models for violence prevention. *Trauma Surgery & Acute Care Open, 9*(1), e001483.

Zavattaro, S. M., Schuneman, C., & Mastracci, S. H. (2024). "Every day of your life you deal with death:" Incorporating dirty work into the MPA curriculum. *Journal of Public Affairs Education, 30*(2), 194–215.

Chapter 11
Practice

Introduction

As a social work student, I was always prone to reading scholarly material with immediate practice implications when all was said and done. Mind you, theoretical and research material were of significant importance. However, the ultimate "so what" question always entered prominently into my thinking in my desire to make an immediate difference in people's lives. I imagine that there are more than a few readers who share this stance. Research and scholarship, as addressed in the previous two chapters and throughout this book, set an important requisite foundation for interventions and education. Research and education, as noted, are a form of intervention. However, we rarely think of them as such. This final chapter will address what most readers think of what constitutes "intervention."

Yes, we have finally arrived at the final chapter! I hope that readers have started to think about how they can best address the death care sector by taking into account their neighborhood's characteristics. There are numerous options that are possible, as described in other parts of this book and evidenced by the high number of interventions discussed in this chapter. These recommendations cover a wide arena, providing sufficient details to grasp the central thrust of the recommendations and also bringing to the fore recommendations related to research and education, which can be viewed as interventions.

Many details will not be covered in order to be more comprehensive due to limited space. The sheer number of practice recommendations reveals how the bottom line is so important, but not intended to diminish the importance of education and research, however. To revisit gun violence statistics again, this nation is facing headwinds. The number of guns manufactured in this country more than doubled from 5.5 million in 2010 to 11 million in 2020, with gun deaths, not unexpectedly, increasing by 43% during this period. Between 2012 and 2022, it increased from

© The Author(s), under exclusive license to Springer Nature Switzerland AG 2025
M. Delgado, *The Death Care Industry and Urban Gun Violence*,
https://doi.org/10.1007/978-3-031-95682-9_11

10.5 to 14.2 deaths per 100,000 people (Schladen, 2024). It does not take a statistician to see that increased availability of guns speaks for itself.

I had to be selective in the number of interventions covered in this chapter because of page limitations and how local circumstances weigh so heavily in how practice can and must unfold, providing a range of interventions necessitating different levels of resources and time commitments. I hope that readers are not expecting a cookie-cutter approach toward death care interventions. Such an approach, not surprisingly, is a disservice to urban communities struggling with the consequences of gun violence.

After all is said and done, it is all about our willingness and ability to take research and training, and the values and principles undergirding these two domains, and converting them into practice. In our case, practice is participatory-centered in highly marginalized urban communities experiencing the worst of gun violence, including this nation's unwillingness to make the necessary changes to prevent gun availability! It is not a leap to think that feelings of despair can lead to actions of despair. These actions compromise communities and their future. Thus, I elected to focus on interventions predicated on varying degrees of commitment and resources to allow local circumstances, budgets, and goals to dictate which ones have a higher probability of achieving success.

Finally, it bears reminding readers that exposure to gun violence brings a wide range of illnesses we do not customarily associate with this violence, such as chronic physical diseases such as heart disease, asthma, stroke, and cancer (Bonne & Dicker, 2020), broadening the practice arena and need for training on gun violence. Consequently, this wide expanse of consequences must limit the type of helping organization for engaging, even when they do not have gun violence as a central focus for their services.

Community Engagement

Readers must not be surprised by my starting with community engagement interventions. Greater understanding of how community violence alters neighborhood interpersonal dynamics is desperately needed in developing strategies (Ross et al., 2021; Stager et al., 2024). Wishing to meaningfully engage all segments of a community in a campaign requires more than the act of wishing, however. It necessitates labor-intensive actions based upon serious deliberations, decisions, and necessary resources.

Community engagement is a serious topic worth the resources and time of conceptualizing what it means. We must endeavor to eschew lumping all urban youth of color in high-violence communities to address a subgroup of gang-involved youth in a rush to provide outreach (Hureau & Papachristos, 2024) and interventions. The same can be said about urban communities since no two are identical.

The concepts of "community participation" and "community input" get bandied about. I had a colleague that would say that there was a significant difference between "grassroots" support and "grass-tips" support. The former is meaningful and labor-intensive; the latter is symbolic. Symbolism is not enough! Meaningful community engagement can easily find a prominent place in the two other chapters in this section, but I decided to lodge it more prominently in this section on practice. Simply stated, "meaningful" translates into hard work and a long-term commitment!

It is no mistake that I started this chapter with a recommendation on participation because of its significance in a community intervention with any hope of achieving success. Readers will never be at a loss encountering community and organizational collaborative models of various types. A fundamental point in examining these models is what seat at the table community representatives will occupy. At one end are the invitees and their assigned seats. At the other end of this continuum are those at the head of the table, dictating how community needs are conceptualized and exploring various ways to meet these needs. This is the stance that I like. Yes, "professionals" have many options that we can propose, so it isn't that we are mere guests and grateful to be invited. As we prove ourselves, and a community grows to know and trust us, we will find our advice more welcomed and solicited when needed. This still makes us guests!

I seriously doubt that I can attend any public forum on gun violence without the subject of community participation being raised. I, too, am a firm believer in community participation and community decision-making, but I would be disingenuous if I did not comment on the challenges this engagement brings for us in the academy. We, in this world, live with great privilege as well as great restraints on our time and the constant pressures of producing research grants and corresponding scholarship. When we embrace a multi-layer view of community trauma, for example, and attempt to fit this worldview within an academic timeline, we are doomed to fail or, at best, come up with a very limited view of what constitutes community trauma (Everytown Research, 2021):

> The ripple effects of community trauma also contribute to fraying the bonds of community cooperation and solidarity. As communities face high levels of trauma, cohesion can break down and trust can erode. This results in such changes as neighbors being less likely to intervene when trouble crops up. When this happens, the community loses the essential 'eyes on the street,' the informal involvement of adults that contributes to safer communities. And this community trauma can dampen residents' capacity and willingness to participate in efforts to develop solutions. In this way, community trauma can hamper the ability of neighbors to work together to address the causes of trauma and build safer communities.

Everytown's perspective matches my experiences with community engagement. Meaningful engagement takes time and significant effort to go along with an expectation that communities will test us. Are we there on a temporary basis until our grant runs out, or are we there for the duration, regardless of funding commitment? With exceptions, most of us do not live in the community we wish to aid. Thus, our viewpoint is limited, necessitating seeking wiser residents to guide us in our work. That is a reality of being community outsiders.

Community engagement can go by a variety of terms, with volunteerism probably being the most well-known, but it must be inclusive to maximize its potential to achieve community healing (Sandberg et al., 2024, p.805): "The practical implications of the current study show that volunteering occupies an important place in community healing and thus deserves to be acknowledged and supported by community leaders." The difference between commissioning a memorial mural and having community members paint a mural is the difference between night and day. Both efforts involve leaving a mark for the community. However, when a mural is painted by the community, the status ascends in significance in helping participants and the community heal (Delgado, 2003).

Meaningful engagement of community is an expanding practice horizon (Francis, 2018). Felter et al. (2023) advance a novel empowerment approach with youth acting as "trauma ambassadors" based on an East North Philadelphia intervention. It is a community-university project that views youth as assets rather than assuming victim roles. Implementation and outcomes of the trauma ambassadors program is a case study of trauma-informed youth leadership development, introducing a prototype of what is possible when we are creative. We must not forget that young people (15–34 years old) are responsible for half of all homicides, with those of color and urban-based more likely to experience and perpetrate this violence (Ross et al., 2024). Logic dictates that any model for an intervention strategy needs to prioritize this age group.

It may seem unnecessary to say. However, how community participation is conceptualized and implemented is dictated by local communities. Communities with high percentages of undocumented residents present different challenges when compared to urban residents of color representing multiple generations within the community and who are citizens. Of course, most urban communities will have a combination of both, including various levels of acculturation. Localities are never the same. Where there is overlap and uniqueness will be influential in shaping interventions. Community engagement can be conceptualized as the "glue" that brings together research and education.

Bridging the Academic and Practice Worlds

A book on death must walk on very tender or sacred ground, and particularly one on gun violence because of how it touches so many lives, including this author, in the interest of self-disclosure. This is particularly more so in high-violence communities, where daily activities become much more difficult to navigate. It seems as if these communities have a daily reminder of those lost to guns and those surviving doing so with complex physical and emotional scars. Opening the field of death care to join in the fight against gun violence, I believe, is a critical element that has yet to be explored in a systematic manner. Gun violence needs "all hands on deck" and cannot afford to have any segment of the community absent from this goal.

Bridging the academic world with the "real" world necessitates walking a careful path that makes sure justice is done to both of these worlds. Closing the gap between these two realms is the "magic spot" in finding solutions that meet the needs of communities in real time, with long-term benefits. These solutions should have immediate and long-term benefits. Low-resourced families and communities often get confronted with an unexpected death, and when discussing guns, one that often leaves the deceased in a physical condition that may render them unrecognizable to loved ones; this is particularly the case with young children because of their size.

Urban community practice's future is only limited by our imagination and willingness to "push the envelope" on behalf of the most vulnerable in our society, opening up new, exciting, and even more challenging possibilities of collaboration. The academy has an important role to play in shaping this field of practice, but again, it must be undertaken in collaboration with the community and sectors new to our vision of what constitutes practice. Further, the academy must reach out across the nation and even internationally in seeking new approaches to solving a major public health problem in this country, even though we occupy a unique position regarding gun violence.

Efforts to bridge the divide between the "real" world and the "academic" world can vary according to intensity. We in the classroom can have outside speakers from the death care sector come and speak in our classes or be part of conferences that we sponsor. In social work, where we rely upon field placements, we can have them in community settings that facilitate part of their placement experiences being in funeral homes or houses of worship, for example. Development of coalitions is labor intensive, and carrying out the establishment of one on gun violence, for instance, can be part of a student's field assignment. Clearly, there is tremendous flexibility in how we bridge the academic and practice arenas.

The frontier of community practice, in turn, will be shaped by today's urban practitioner's vision, embracing the rewards as well as the challenges, some anticipated and others unanticipated. The greater the challenge, then the greater the potential outcomes and rewards. This future is predicated on having practitioners be prepared to dare envision this future and embrace new research and intervention possibilities. Entering the world of the urban death care sector and gun violence is such an example! In many ways, it is a new world awaiting us, and we must embrace the moment. It has unimaginable benefits for communities if we dare to venture into uncharted territory.

Churches and Gun Violence Initiatives

Houses of worship interested in saving the souls and the bodies of parishioners will find themselves aiding their communities, too. Black churches, for example, can ascend to leading community efforts to fight oppression, and seeking voting rights is as old as the institution itself. That stance only served to enhance their reputation and influence within the Black community, drawing on their critical role during the civil rights era. This institution stands high on unparalleled and unchallenged moral ground. Nevertheless, it still can be the subject of gun violence even when occupying an exalted position. That makes violence within their midst that much more significant from a community standpoint.

Obviously, the fight against gun violence is not a new idea in Boston and other cities, and that is well documented in the scholarly literature. Spirituality among Black-American men who have been injured through gun violence, for instance, has slowly entered the domain of being conceptualized as a key social determinant of health (Ransome, 2020). Although spirituality is not the exclusive domain of religious institutions, the Black Church is well positioned to foster its use by helping to address the trauma that guns cause.

In fact, Black churches can be valuable sources of collective efficacy. They are morally and strategically well positioned to mobilize other religious institutions in addition to community organizations (traditional and non-traditional) and residents of all ages because guns impact all age groups. In gist, you do not have to be a direct victim to be impacted!

Faith-based interventions focused on second victims, for example, illustrate the role and importance of these institutes by uplifting activities that bring medical-religious partners together in pursuit of a greater understanding of how to better research and serve these victims. Probably more importantly, it demonstrates the crossing of spheres and professions in playing a more informed and active role in addressing the varied ramifications of gun violence, opening the door for other efforts.

Houses of worship are caught up in community gun violence, becoming more frequent crime scenes for this type of violence. However, shootings at churches, mosques, temples, and cemeteries are not unique to this country. We only have to travel back in time to 1988, when 3 people were killed and 50 wounded at a Belfast cemetery in Northern Ireland. This holy site was selected to maximize casualties and send a powerful political message, not too dissimilar to what happens in the case of the United States; it often involves gang-related activities, although the ones that are politically motivated gain the greater national attention.

The following declarative statement by Congressional Representative Brown (2024) uplifts how shootings in places once considered sacred feed into feelings of defeatism and despair that are far-reaching into the "soul of a community," if not the nation:

> Imagine being in church for the funeral of a gun violence victim and hearing shots going off outside. That was my experience late last year and it summed up how overwhelmed this country is by gun violence, building mountains of despair with tragedy after tragedy. This past December, I attended the celebration of life service for Di'Mesha Wright, when it was interrupted by gunfire. Twenty-three-year-old Di'Mesha was killed by a shooter using an AR-style rifle to shoot through the front door of a home. Di'Mesha was holding her 7-month-old baby when she was shot. As we gathered to remember her and pray for her family, we heard shots ring out. People ran from the aisles and sought cover. And an already painful day was made even worse.

Losing sacred sites to gun violence creates a level of despair new to communities historically accustomed to facing a variety of challenges to health and well-being. Breaching sites considered "off-limits" or "sacred" signals an evolutionary leap and the need for radically reconceptualizing "the war on guns" and what that really means. This calls for bold initiatives seeking and metaphors to match the challenge and a shift in paradigms. Houses of worship and clergy have assumed more prominent positions initiating programs and actions on urban gun violence in service to their congregations and communities. The following are two such examples, out of the countless—one based in New York City and the other in Atlanta, Georgia—typifying these new ventures that can serve as models for other cities.

The gun violence field desperately needs innovative models with implications for other cities, big, medium, or small, across the country. It is not a practice field that we can easily turn to the international scene for new practice models because of the prominence and nature of gun ownership in this country and our willingness to engage in gun violence to settle disputes, real or imagined. I am afraid to say gun violence is as American as it can get, taking its place alongside hot dogs and apple pies.

In 2024, New York City launched a high-profile three-pronged initiative titled "Citywide Clergy Coalition," with state funding supporting a coordinated anti-gun violence intervention through clergy leadership and involvement (New York City, 2024):

> **Street-Level Engagement:** Increasing and expanding community engagement through clergy walks, street dinners, arts, sports, mentorship, and hotspots programs. **Victim Support Services:** Increasing private support of families and survivors of gun violence through prayer vigils, bereavement services, transportation, emergency accommodations, food, and spiritual care. **Precinct Engagement:** Connecting with local precincts to support young people with criminal backgrounds, bolstering anti-violence groups, and working with community stakeholders.

This multi-pronged approach acknowledges the need for a broad intervention strategy to be inclusive of all demographic segments, with youth ascending in importance to occupy positions with authority rather than merely being representative of this group. Youth and young adults disproportionately bear a tremendous burden in gun violence in New York City and throughout the nation.

Also in 2024, Atlanta launched their version of a clergy initiative to create safe spaces and provide needed support for other services to eliminate gun violence (Mack, 2024). Initiatives such as these are needed but specifically tailored to funeral homes and other death-related service providers, in addition to taking into consideration public spaces.

Where are the major initiatives involving the death care industry? The answer is that they are still in their infancy, and I am being kind. However, a "big tent" umbrella can effectively incorporate these businesses, with each sector, or spoke, receiving due attention that takes into account their unique positions and responsibilities. Other cities have initiated coalitions with clergy actively leading gun violence initiatives. Baltimore, for example, initiated a gang prevention program for church leaders. The PAGE (Pastors against Gangs Everywhere) initiative seeks engagement of church leaders to offer afterschool programs to deter at-risk youth from joining gangs, a key factor in that city's crime and gun violence rates. Houses of worship are often integral to the functioning of urban communities, and they must have a seat at the table in helping to localize interventions, as evidenced in this section.

"Final Words" Matter: Black/Latino Youth Writing Their Own Obituaries

This recommendation will receive greater depth of coverage than the other recommendations in this chapter due to its significance and the challenges it will present practitioners. On the initial view, this practice recommendation may seem odd to the typical reader, and that is understandable. Obituaries symbolize a final act of saying goodbye and how we want the deceased to be remembered. So much is anticipated during the final moments before we put a loved one to rest. In fact, I venture to guess that few readers have even gone to the point of selecting and ordering the final themes that they want to leave for attendees at a last rites ceremony.

It is worth spending a few moments in grounding multiple ways for tapping the voices of residents prior to covering the writing of obituaries. Nickerson (2024) describes the use of letter writing in addressing trauma and Black women, which can be adopted for use with gun violence, such as writing a letter to one's family sharing their thoughts, aspirations, and how they want to be remembered, for example. Other methods, of course, can be used, such as videos, artwork, photovoice (Counselman-Carpenter, 2024), or other communicative means that take into account project goals, funding, and circumstances such as siblings killed as the focus. The central goals, however, remain the same in helping participants deal with trauma.

I wonder how many readers have even thought about their own obituary, let alone written a draft of one. I certainly have not, if any reader is interested in knowing! The exercise of writing one's own obituary can result in reflections that engender the importance of striving to become a better self (Payne et al., 2022), bringing a positive outcome for participants. Many of us grew up reading them in the local newspaper, providing the public a brief glimpse into the life of someone. They are never too long but long enough to provide a snapshot of their lives and why they would be missed. These individuals generally hold an esteemed position within a city, with some degree of recognition by the general public. I never could relate to these writings in my neighborhood of the South Bronx, New York. However, I knew about their existence and general importance.

Some readers, as already noted, may view the writing of one's own obituary as unthinkable or even morbid, particularly for youth who potentially have multiple decades of life ahead of them. However, the subject of writing one's own obituary is gaining popularity, as evidenced by any Google search on the subject, particularly if we wish to leave lasting impressions of loved ones to the general public. The writing of one's own obituary and the structured discussion that follows with others in a group undertaking this task, for example, can help participants share their concerns in a manner that has relevance to their surroundings, such as youth of color who have experienced the death of close ones due to guns. Most importantly, when done with a group, it helps participants to see that they are not alone with their dreams and despairs.

Helping those with non-therapeutic grieving is often associated with violent and unexpected deaths, and for those lucky to survive these shootings, it is potentially leading to severe emotional distress that may go unrecognized by authorities and therefore untreated. Early in this book, I uplifted the importance of storytelling. This form of narrative is generally not about oneself. How best to help urban youth, in turn, requires innovative approaches to tap these voices, including using social media, as highlighted in this book.

Participants can share their hopes and fears, including how they may be viewed by others left behind. Leading these discussions takes on significant importance in helping them identify themes of how they have been traumatized by gun violence, including the strategies that can be successful in avoiding contentious situations that can lead to gun violence. Further, effective strategies and tactics, too, can be shared, bringing greater significance to group members.

Rynearson and Salloum (2021, p.177) put a spotlight on the significance of "restorative retelling" for helping those with prolonged grief after a violent death or traumatic circumstances: "The goal of restorative retelling is to revise the narrative memory of reenactment through a collaborative, corrective retelling, so that in its modified form the memory remains but no longer demands reenactment and restitution." Accomplishing this goal, of course, is notable but also arduous without expert guidance and corresponding instrumental and expressive support.

Self-help groups, often led by mothers of children killed by guns, for example, have emerged to aid families of victims with similar gun violence experiences through concrete and emotional help (Delgado, 2021). Helping those with non-therapeutic grieving is often associated with violent and unexpected deaths and potentially leading to severe emotional distress that can often go unreported and untreated for fear of stigma. How best to help these individuals, in turn, requires innovative and localized approaches.

Self-help groups can be an excellent locally based mechanism for undertaking what Rynearson and Salloum (2021, p.177) call "restorative retelling," for example, putting a spotlight on the significance of retelling to help those with prolonged grief after a violent death: "The goal of restorative retelling is to revise the narrative memory of reenactment through a collaborative, corrective retelling, so that in its modified form the memory remains but no longer demands reenactment and restitution."

Durham, North Carolina, for example, initiated a restorative justice program titled "*Listening to Survivors of Gun Violence*" (2023) focused on 17-year-old or older survivors and loved ones and involved a collaboration between public, private, and community partners. This initiative was built upon a series of structured listening meetings co-led by a two-person team consisting of a trained community facilitator and a survivor of gun violence or a loved one of a victim (Restorative Justice, 2023, p.15): "One of the most important lessons learned from the P4R project is the inherent value of listening to survivors of gun violence using a non-judgmental narrative process. Almost all participants expressed gratitude for the program, with the program formative for participants to rebuild their social skills following the original trauma. Although our program facilitators were not practicing therapists, this program attests to the therapeutic nature of a structured listening program for people impacted by gun violence."

Imaginative readers can see the potential of a restorative justice centered project (Rice et al., 2024) to help communities in their recovery process. These types of interventions, of course, can be tailored to gun violence in any particular locale, because place and space influence how shooting events are experienced. To the best of my knowledge, this type of intervention has not been attempted to reach those who experienced gun violence during a last rites ceremony to have them share this very particular and personal experience, which is increasingly finding relevance across the nation's cities.

This new arena would be representative of projects that can be initiated to specifically tap into gun violence's consequences in the death care sector. Modifications to a standard approach, of course, can be made to take into account the unique circumstances that will be encountered. However, one dimension of community trauma that bears spotlighting is how Black-American and Brown youth think about their own deaths. "Deaths of despair," signifying an end-of-life due to factors out of to our own control ((Deaton & Case, 2020, p.38): "an epidemic that is not carried by a virus or a bacterium, nor is it caused by an external agent, such as poisoning of the air or the fallout from a nuclear accident, instead, people are doing this to themselves."

These deaths are generally due to suicides, drug overdoses, and liver disease from alcohol abuse. Gun violence, other than self-inflicted, can fall under this category, as in the case of this book. I would take the liberty of including gun violence and the emotional toll it takes when done at the hands of others sharing the same community and socio-economic circumstances (Gross, 2020). As an aside, I was surprised that after an extensive review of the popular and scholarly literature, and outreach to colleagues across the country, I could not locate a single source of material on this topic. It is an exercise that I have used with youth of color and found it profoundly helpful in having them share their vision for how they expect to die but also, just as importantly, be remembered.

Sadly, the vast majority of these youth saw themselves dying young and not in older adulthood, with gun violence the primary method of causing their deaths. Not one said that they would live to a ripe old age and die of natural causes. I venture to guess that if I were to go to an economically privileged community and did the same exercise that I would find similar results! It may seem unthinkable for youth of any background to anticipate their own deaths and how they will be viewed by loved ones and friends, particularly since they have their whole life ahead of them.

However, that is a realty that is before us. How does a 10-year-old, for example, fathom the end of life even when death surrounds them?

Seeking mental health services in acute situations, for example, where it may be expected to have someone call 911, is not a viable option in many urban neighborhoods because of fears of being killed by the police (Price et al., 2021), putting an exclamation point on a tragic situation to begin with in marginalized communities. That may be difficult for some readers to fathom. However, the stressors of knowing that once we leave home that there are minefields in our surroundings, translates into a keen awareness, with all of the emotional or psychic energy it takes, of how life can be cut short at a second in time and not being able to say goodbyes to our loved ones; they, in turn, could not say their goodbyes, too. This makes final rites at a critical event in the eyes of those left behind. To soil that moment, so to speak, makes a tragedy even more difficult to comprehend and heal from, too.

Community Safe Spaces for Healing

Any meaningful review of the gun violence literature will find constant mention of the importance of "safe spaces" for healing to transpire in helping victims of trauma recover. These spaces can assume to occupy different settings and circumstances (Grant et al., 2023), such as houses of worship and self-help organizations, for example.

Safe spaces, of course, can be conceptualized in a variety of ways to take into account local circumstances. The emergence of Death Cafes, for instance, although not specific to gun-related deaths, represent an effort to designate spaces for attendees to engage in meaningful, culturally relevant, and often arduous have meaningful and difficult conversations about death and dying (Cherry & Black, 2024). Spaces with similar goals can be developed within established institutions such as funeral parlors and houses of worship, for instance.

Nevertheless, regardless of setting and locale, safe spaces are in short supply in high violence communities and must account for local circumstances pertaining to language, cultural factors, and accessibility—geographical, cultural/linguistic, operational (days and times), and most importantly, psychological—namely, non-stigmatizing. Readers will see these themes in this section and should feel free to be creative in thinking about the circumstances that they find themselves within to create safe spaces to meet their needs.

Healing safe spaces are in great demand and essential (Moreno et al., 2024; Walker et al., 2024). There is a universal longing for these spaces in communities of color. Surprisingly, these spaces sometimes organically appear out of nowhere and at other times they must be purposely created. These spaces allow attendees to meet others facing many of the same challenges. Residents of high gun violence neighborhoods need to be able to share their hurt, obtain validation, and just as importantly, to know that they are not alone. They can be themselves and be able to use the language of their choice, which has cultural concepts that have meaning for them.

Herford (2023) speaks to the importance of creating sanctuary for those called "tragically bereaved," capturing the degree of sadness that accompanies this situation, with a list of seven actions that increase the likelihood of achieving a healthy state of mind:

> 1. Suspend our judgments about grief; 2. Pay close attention to the people around us: listen for what they say and don't say; speak up if we notice a change in their appetite, sleep, or accessibility; 3. Prioritize connection in your community as a lifesaving measure; 4. Ask the scary questions and make space for difficult answers; 5. Confront our helplessness and take action anyway; 6. Employ radical empathy: listen with love, speak with compassion.; and 7. Pause and offer our full attention and caring presence, over and over again.

As readers can discern from the above list, there is no "magic" one approach solution to this problem. There is a communal approach that increase the likelihood of a therapeutic outcome when we connect with others who have health and well-being in mind. These authors discuss the blurring of the memorialization practices undertaken by community members and death care providers, calling attention to the benefits of the formal and informal worlds coming together.

This partnership, so to speak, is facilitated when the death care sector can also envision their role as educators and facilitators, transcending their traditional roles, allowing the moment to dictate the most therapeutic role to prevail and the local scene dictating the most propitious approach. This allows local circumstances surrounding the death and socio-cultural customs to emerge and take center stage. The moment, in other words, dictates this final farewell.

Bamwine et al.' (2024) study of Pittsburgh Black-American adolescents who lost a family member or friend to gun violence found the importance of them having a safe place and space to share narratives of their loss was instrumental in helping them heal and experience post-traumatic growth. Mind you, I am cognizant that these safe spaces may be in short supply in high-violence neighborhoods. The funeral homes where they attended to pay their last respects, for example, can serve as places where these types of groups can meet. Such actions on the part of a funeral parlor will further integrate them into a community's social fabric. Trauma care providers can co-lead these discussion groups, for example.

Funeral homes, it bears mentioning, have the physical space for these gatherings to occur and are often geographically easily accessible because of their community location. Readers may rightly raise the potential of stigma associated with meeting in these spaces needing to be addressed, which will vary according to community histories and relationships with these institutions. Readers may initially resist such an approach. However, the community will show less resistance than us. Ascending to this healing role, however, may make funeral homes more likely to be targets of retribution!

We cannot allow gun violence voices at a last rites ceremony to go without specific attention to their unique experience because failure to recognize their experience can lead to further emotional consequences. The initiative or program can be modified according to the circumstances of the local community experience and budgets. Readers are able to use their imagination in accomplishing this task.

Safe spaces bring universal qualities that allow for different forms of programming to emerge taking into account local circumstances and interests. The use of drama therapy to address trauma has started to gain currency as part of an expanding terrain of interventions that go beyond conventional talk therapy and illustrative of the potential for gun-related trauma. Not surprisingly, this intervention relies on having a safe space. Drama therapy, of course, also necessitates that it is grounded within cultural affirming spaces (Black et al., 2024). Arts-based trauma-Informed approaches, too, fall within this realm (Porter, 2024). Musical theater is yet another form of community engagement project helping to engage communities in addressing trauma for those inclined to this form of performance art (Windle, 2024).

Opportunities for survivors of gun violence at final rites events to systematically share their experiences in a formalized way are very limited, even when they return home and have a need to talk and share about what transpired. There is no place and space for this to transpire in an organized manner. These shooting experiences are very unique and are probably best understood by others who have experienced them. The intervention to be described did not involve shootings at a death rite event but can be tailored to those with this form of violence.

The absence of safe spaces makes it arduous to grow and prosper, effectively undermining our roles within families and communities. That stance should not come as any great surprise to readers. This topic permeates all forms of interventions but takes on greater saliency when discussing gun violence.

Involvement of Black and Latino Religious Institutions in Community Coalitions

If you ever have an opportunity to talk with a social worker who is a community activist, you will invariably hear the word "coalition." In this case, it is a recommendation of a coalition of gun violence activists. However, I am calling on the religious sector to create local coalitions to address gun violence, particularly in neighborhoods enduring the greatest consequences of this violence. Various examples were highlighted throughout this book. Providing needed support to community initiatives will invariably necessitate the involvement of the religious sector. Religious leaders must garner institutional resources beyond providing space for meetings.

Addressing neighborhood gun violence can also translate into making houses of worship safer for all attendees, including religious leadership, as highlighted in this book. Houses of worship can be conceptualized as beacons of light ("pathways") during stormy times, providing safe spaces for those in pain and in need.

There is no magical number of participants to make a coalition. In fact, it may start very small, and with time, visibility, and success, expand in the number of participants/organizations. Participating in these coalitions does not preclude participation in other coalitions, which is typical based on my experiences in the field. Gun violence, it bears noting, intersects with countless other community issues. Engaging in coalitions allows for varying degrees of time and resource commitments. Having youth participate in these coalitions, however, should be a priority. Having houses of worship play prominent roles in these initiatives will prove to bring many benefits as well as challenges, too!

Cadre of Community Mentors

Forming a cadre of community mentors that can be deployed (emergency response team) at a moment's notice is critical to not only helping families grieve but also possibly limiting the escalation of violence. Community mentors are often strategically situated to aid youth in coping with concerns about safety and the emotional toll that community violence extracts (Byrd et al., 2024). Identifying and supporting these mentors can help bridge the divide youth of color often encounter, particularly in coping with gun violence and resulting deaths of peers and loved ones.

High gun violence communities have outstanding residents who able to serve as community mentors for those in great pain, as in the case of East St. Louis, Ill.'s Roby-Bell: "When April Roby-Bell joined the Gangster Disciples in middle school, the street gang treated her like family when she felt abandoned by her own. She was looking for love, acceptance, and stability. 'They trained us as little kids. How to own your 'hood, own your street: 'This is my territory,'" Roby-Bell said. The experience also taught her tough lessons about life and death at an early age. At least half of the friends she grew up with are now dead. "At times, it became hard because you just get tired of fighting," she said. "I probably should have been dead a long time ago." There is guilt in being a survivor that can linger on throughout life, serving as a key motivator to give back in whatever way possible. Roby-Bell is a pillar of virtue and strength for others, offering advice, planning, and presiding over funerals of strangers and friends.

Community-driven interventions can be group-specific, as in the case of Black women who have experienced a traumatic loss, and can also be highly viable in crafting trauma-informed interventions that take into account local circumstances (Castelin et al., 2024). These same members, in turn, can also assume mentor roles, reflecting the wide flexibility that community residents can assume based upon their abilities and willingness to engage in multiple roles.

Formal systems of care will do well by identifying, enlisting, and supporting community informal mentors. These mentors can exist throughout a community, including the death care sector, helping to bridge formal with informal services when trusted by both sides, making them invaluable in any gun violence initiative. Just as importantly, interacting with them is non-stigmatizing, a key consideration in communities fearful of being labeled as having emotional problems. These individuals are not meant to replace formally trained therapists. They can, for example, facilitate referrals and break down potential barriers to accessing needed care.

These mentors, of course, are not limited to serving youth but can help adults, too. These individuals may be part of existing service structures within a community. Because of their personal experiences and training, they are uniquely positioned to address the needs emanating from gun violence at final rites events. Community organizations can make these individuals available when needed. When not needed, they can continue to perform their usual duties. It reminds me of how a volunteer fire department functions for readers having difficulty in conceptualizing this role.

Community mentors exist to address a wide variety of local social problems. The gun violence field is no exception. Having community mentors break down stereotypes about the death care sector can have a prominent place in a constellation of community-centered interventions.

Lack of Justice: A Troubling Picture

Although the subject of the justice system was specifically addressed in Chap. 10, it is too important to not address again. Where is the justice system? This question is not meant to be provocative but really practical in nature. If the families of dead victims believe that the perpetrators of violence can do so with impunity and the justice system is ineffectual, at best, in bringing them to justice, then they must take justice into their own hands. There is no question that there often is a community justice system that can only feed into violence. If our justice system is negligent, to be polite, then justice falls into the hands of residents to carry out. Their existence, not surprisingly, can be problematic, undermining the formal justice system (Ahmad & Von Wangenheim, 2021).

Urban communities, some of which have high national profiles and have experienced exceptional levels of gun fatalities, do not have much confidence in the police and the judicial system based upon treatment in the past, and statistics do bear this stance out because of low clearance (arrests and adjudication) crime rates. Only 20% of fatal shootings result in an arrest, for example, let alone convictions and sentences to prison (Oceguera & Agrelo, 2023).

This "lack of justice" is not lost in high-violence communities, further compounding the grieving and healing process for families. An interrupted grieving process because of a lack of justice does not spell well for those who grieve as they seek to move forward with their lives. Lack of professional help for families, in turn, leaves a long-lasting scar that shapes their daily interactions and engenders fears of further gun violence continuing unabated.

One parent stated it well concerning the mother of Zaire, a shooting fatality with relevance to the rest of the United States: "Grief comes in waves," she said. "One minute you're doing kind of OK, and then the next, you're crying and sick to your stomach." "Constantly thinking of Zaire being gone is a mental drain," she said. "We're in a club we didn't ask to be in," Nelson said. "It is a space that is constantly growing in Chicago." Misery, simply stated, does not welcome company. The arrest and sentencing of a culprit does not bring back the deceased. It does allow grieving families and their families a sense of justice prevailing, which is a critical component of a journey toward healing; the loved ones of the perpetrator, in turn, will experience grief. There is simply no escaping grief for families and neighborhoods.

A feeling that justice cannot be expected unless we take it into our own hands is troubling. The police and the court system must be a part of any comprehensive effort at addressing gun violence. Bridging divides, as in the case of the death care system, will aid communities in the short and long term, although not without acknowledging the challenges that these efforts will bring.

Final Comments for Readers

One of my earliest memories of attending a burial ceremony was for my uncle during my fifth grade. The amount of crying and emotions at that burial was intense. There were even attempts of family members being restrained from throwing themselves into the grave and having to be held back by attendees. I learned that this intensity in the show of emotion was expected to show how much they loved and would miss the deceased. Experiencing gunfire on that occasion would have left me with an even greater life-altering emotional reaction, one that would have altered my DNA if that were possible. Funeral rites for people of color in marginalized communities are sacred and produce lifetime memories that only get compromised by gunfire!

Experiencing gun violence has far outpaced experiencing opportunities for advancement and well-being in countless urban undervalued communities, and that is such a sad commentary in this country with a reputation that the sky is the limit in privileged communities. Life is open to so many countless potential possibilities. However, being a victim of gun violence is not one that many of us aspire to achieve. The future contributions of those killed will be forever lost to their families, communities, and the nation.

There were several instances during the writing of this book that I shared personal comments with readers. That is not unusual for me if there are any new readers of my writings. This will be the last time, for what it is worth. In a moment of self-disclosure, I have had a close relative killed by gun violence; I have also had a close relative take the life of another because of gun violence and be sentenced to prison. I have had close friends survive gun violence to tell the tale and walk around with bullet scars and fragments in their body as a constant reminder of that encounter. Those images and stories stay with you for a lifetime. Why self-disclose? Readers probably picked up that authoring this book is so much more than a "scholarly pursuit" to advance the field.

This book is about helping those who struggle on a daily basis to deal with the guilt that often emerges about not doing more about preventing gun violence. There simply isn't enough funding, practice, and research being conducted on what many people consider to be a major public health challenge in this country, and more specifically its core urban centers. We must move to help individuals so that we do not forget about the broader neighborhood or community.

These two perspectives must be present in order to help each other. The magnitude of the ramifications of gun violence is too enormous to just concentrate on one avenue. The community trauma avenue has been neglected for too long. This road must be expansive enough to include the death care sector to help communities in the long road to recovery, in addition to stopping this form of violence. I have had to be an optimist by nature and believe as the field expands its vision, we will get there.

It may seem as if re-traumatization in high gun violence communities is a daily reality, making successful recovery that much more difficult to achieve. Repeated gun violence does not provide residents with the space and time from which recovery can be initiated and sustained, thus requiring us to think of this condition from a community trauma standpoint. This form of recovery is predicated on group and neighborhood activities that provide us with therapeutic spaces, sometimes referred to as sanctuaries (Herford, 2023).

On a more personal note, the journey of authoring a book is an adventure that never conforms to expectations or gets old, so to speak. I guess what we can say that about is life itself. My journey in authoring this book was guided by what I thought was a clear destination as outlined in the section on goals. This journey is one of discovery for me, too, which is an experience that is always personally rewarding and I never tire of. There were "high" and "low" moments, as to be expected, particularly when writing about lives lost before their time, such as in the case of children and the aftermath that awaits those left behind and their challenges in moving forward. However, the extent of the challenge was more complex than expected. The Supreme Court decision to allow bump stocks, for example, was such an example.

The gun violence field will never be at a loss for conceptualizing this form of violence. There is no disputing, for example, that gun violence is clustered along time and space dimensions (Weisburd et al., 2012). The same can be said for place (Knorre & MacDonald, 2023). Boston, for instance, over a 29-year period, witnessed gun violence occurring in only 11.5% of its street segments (Braga et al., 2010). That means that almost 90% of that city does not have to worry about being shot! The venture of viewing gun violence within cemeteries, funeral homes, and houses of worship is but the latest expansion of this argument and illustrative of the reach of gun violence in all facets of our lives, including when we die or pay respects.

Destroying cemeteries during genocidal campaigns represents one extreme form of perpetrating violence on the dead and those who still remember and loved those buried there (Krikler, 2023). When we conceptualize urban cemeteries as extensions of specific neighborhoods (Raudon, 2023), it requires thinking of crime (gun violence and vandalism of gravestones) at these settings as part of neighborhood violence, although the scholarly literature has not made this linkage. Thinking of cemeteries as part of the "hood," so to speak, makes it easier to rationalize thinking of burial spaces and places as extensions of the neighborhood and fair game for the execution of violence.

We do not have the luxury of keeping away law enforcement in cases where a burial can be expected to cause a violent reaction that can involve guns; thus the police must be involved in decreasing the odds that violence will ensue at a burial event. A key question is how to implement their involvement in a manner that maintains safety with a minimal visible profile to ensure that the dignity of a final rites ceremony is not compromised.

I make this recommendation cognizant of the range of intense responses that it may elicit, particularly in communities with long histories of distrust and tensions with law enforcement. However, families in grief are not in the best state of mind or position to exercise sound judgment and maintain peace at a final rites ceremony. The frequency of funeral shootings has dramatically increased and raised sufficient alarm to have localities call for special task forces, including the police, to address this problem in a systemic manner because the death care sector cannot handle the violence without external help (Inklebarger, 2018):

> Johnson (Director of Smith & Thomas Funeral Home in Maywood, Illinois) and others say the processions are made even more dangerous when they involve the death of a slain gang member. Law enforcement officials have dubbed them 'rowdy processions'—many of which pass through Oak Park and Forest Park along Roosevelt Road and Jackson Boulevard—because of gang members blocking traffic, threatening other motorists, hanging out of car windows and, in some cases, firing weapons... The frequency of such dangerous processions has increased over the last few years, prompting the Cook County Board of Commissioners to establish a task force to find ways to reduce the trend. Those in the so-called 'death care' industry are also looking for solutions to keep their staff and patrons safe, but they worry that the effort could result in fines and increased regulatory burdens for funeral home operations.

This problem is national in scope, calling for a national summit and solutions rather than letting local municipalities create interventions. I think an equivalent example is dealing with car-related deaths locally rather than nationally in making cars safer. A patchwork of policies and actions does not serve the public interest in the short and long run.

However, saying goodbyes is a multi-step process. The customary cultural practice of having a funeral procession drive by the home of the deceased may not be possible because it entails entering a designated gang territory, including the spot where the deceased was killed. This "compromise" may seem minor for some readers, but it can be far from that when a family has had the misfortune of losing several members to gun violence in their neighborhood. The symbolic "Not Welcomed" sign may be just too much to bear for these families.

Conclusion

This chapter highlighted how open the field of gun violence is for innovative approaches to addressing the death care field in helping urban communities struggling with gun violence during this critical stage of the lifecycle. I noted in the introductory chapter that I needed to capture the reader's attention. I only hope that you have made it this far in your journey! The rationale for recommendations in the final three chapters has roots throughout earlier portions of this book.

Helping professions and academics can no longer ignore the death care sector. In fact, society can no longer ignore and take for granted these services if we hope to remain a viable society, allowing families and loved ones to pay their final respects in a safe and affirming environment! Some readers may think of this declarative statement as hyperbole. Death is a component of the lifecycle, lest we forget that. If that stage is neglected, we will all suffer. The gun violence field must expand its scope regarding who should be a part of these efforts in collaboration with communities, with all of the rewards and challenges it brings.

References

Ahmad, J., & Von Wangenheim, G. (2021). Access to justice: An evaluation of the informal justice systems. *Liberal Arts and Social Sciences International Journal (LASSIJ), 5*(1), 228–244.

Bamwine, P. M., Wallace, J. M., Jaime, M. C. D., Morrow, S. E., Booth, J., & Miller, E. (2024). Exploring bereavement processes among BLACK adolescent male CO-VICTIMS of homicide. *Social Science & Medicine, 352*, 116997.

Black, C., Frederico, M., & Bamblett, M. (2024). 'Healing through culture': Aboriginal young people's experiences of social and emotional wellbeing impacts of cultural strengthening programs. *Child Abuse & Neglect, 148*, 106206.

Bonne, S., & Dicker, R. A. (2020). Hospital-based violence intervention programs to address social determinants of health and violence. *Current Trauma Reports, 6*, 23–28.

Braga, A. A., Papachristos, A. V., & Hureau, D. M. (2010). The concentration and stability of gun violence at micro places in Boston, 1980–2008. *Journal of Quantitative Criminology, 26*, 33–53.

Byrd, K. A., Lohrmann, D. K., Obeng, C., Agley, J., Cate, B., Wong, Y. J., et al. (2024). Coping with community violence: Perspectives of African American young adult men and Hispanic/Latino young adult men. *Journal of Interpersonal Violence, 39*(3–4), 676–706.

Castelin, S., Sáenz Jiménez, A. P., Soto, D., Daniels, L. D., Brown, A. D., & Fehrenbach, T. (2024). Voices that matter: A community-driven intervention framework for Black women who have experienced traumatic loss. *American Journal of Orthopsychiatry*. https://doi.org/10.1037/ort0000771

Cherry, J., & Black, L. W. (2024). "Talking About Funerals Won't Make You Dead": dialogic tensions in death café design and facilitation. *OMEGA-Journal of Death and Dying, 00302228241272716*.

Congressional Representative Brown. (2024, May 4). *To act on gun violence; we have to drop defeatism and despair*. https://pk.headtopics.com/news/to-act-on-gun-violence-we-have-to-drop-defeatism-and-50425896

Counselman-Carpenter, E. (2024). PhotoVoice as a vehicle for promoting posttraumatic growth. In R. Berger (Ed.), *The Routledge international handbook of posttraumatic growth* (pp. 507–516). Routledge.

Deaton, A., & Case, A. (2020). *Deaths of despair and the future of capitalism*. Princeton University Press.

Delgado, M. (2003). *Death at an early age and the urban scene: The case for memorial murals and community healing*. Greenwood Publishing Group.

Delgado, M. (2021). *Urban gun violence: Self-help organizations as healing sites, catalysts for change, and collaborative partnerships*. Oxford University Press.

Everytown Research. (2021). *Invisible wounds: Gun violence and community trauma among Black Americans*. New York.

Felter, J., Chung, H. L., Guth, A., & DiDonato, S. (2023). Implementation and outcomes of the trauma ambassadors program: A case study of trauma-informed youth leadership development. *Child and Adolescent Social Work Journal*, 1–17.

Francis, M. (2018). A narrative inquiry into the experience of being a victim of gun violence. *Journal of Trauma Nursing|JTN, 25*(6), 381–388.

Grant, N., Neville, H., Ogunfemi, N., Smith, A., Groth, S., & Rodriguez, N. (2023). An emerging youth-centered model of community resilience in communities impacted by gun violence: Power through Black Community and Unity. *American Journal of Community Psychology, 71*(3–4), 355–370.

Gross, N. M. N. (2020). *Brothers in grief: The stages of grieving for a school and its students following three shooting deaths of black teenage boys* (Doctoral dissertation, University of Pennsylvania, Philadelphia, PA).

Herford, N. K. (2023, January 9). *Creating sanctury for the tragically bereaved*. https://www.thirteen.org/blog-post/creating-sanctuary-bereaved/

Hureau, D. M., & Papachristos, A. V. (2024). Re-centering the community in violence intervention: Reclaiming legacies of street outreach in the provision of public safety. *Annual Review of Criminology, 8*.

Inklebarger, T. (2018, May 29). Gang burials a problem in western suburbs. County begins work in preparation of new funeral task force. *Forest Park Review*. https://www.forestparkreview.com/2018/05/29/gang-buria-a-problem-in-western-suburbs/

Kirker, N. (2023, May 18). Killing the dead: The logic of cemetery destruction during genocidal campaigns. *Nations and Nationalism, 29*(4), 1338–1354.

Knorre, A., & MacDonald, J. (2023). Shootings and land use. *Journal of Criminal Justice, 86*, 102068.

Mack, E. (2024, April 22). Atlanta faith coalition to seek to curb gun violence. *Fox5Atlanta*. https://www.fox5atlanta.com/news/atlanta-faith-coalition-to-seeks-to-curb-gun-violence

Moreno, F., Dennis, S. H., Cummings, E. M., & Boxer, P. (2024). "When someone is in a safe place, I believe that your mind rests" emotional security amid community violence: A cross-national study with youth in Newark, New Jersey, USA, and San Pedro Sula, Cortés, Honduras. *International Journal of Intercultural Relations, 99*, 101941.

New York City. (2024, January 31). *At annual Interfaith Breakfast, Mayor Adams, Faith Leaders launch citywide cleargy collective to prevent gun violence*. https://www.nyc.gov/office-of-the-mayor/news/086-24/at-annual-interfaith-breakfast-mayoradams-faith-leaders-launch-citywide-clergy-collective-to#/0

Nickerson, B. (2024). *Dear Mama: An exploration of trauma and black feminist healing practices through letter writing*. Scholars Archive. University of Albany State of New York.

Oceguera, R., & Agrelo, J. (2023, December 19). Chicago police make an arrest in only 20 percent of fatal shootings. The failure to solve many of the city's gun crimes has left families distrustful of police and fearful for their own safety. *Hyde Park Herald*. https://www.hpherald.com/evening_digest/chicago-police-make-an-arrest-in-only-20-percent-of-fatal-shootings/article_a1afb5b8-9dcb-11ee-a752-5b206c564929.html

Payne, J., Jones, D., Hwang, J., Babar, H., Tse, E., Mock, K., & Moyer, A. (2022). Writing one's own obituary: Student reflections on an assignment in a positive psychology class. *Journal of Happiness and Health, 2*(2), 98–107.

Porter, J. J. (2024). Complicated grief: An arts-based trauma-informed approach. *Merrimack College.* https://scholarworks.merrimack.edu/cgi/viewcontent.cgi?article=1111&context=soe_student_ce

Price, J. H., Khubchandani, J., & Foh, E. P. (2021). Unintentional firearm mortality in African–American youths, 2010–2019. *Journal of the National Medical Association, 113*(5), 580–586.

Ransome, Y. (2020). Religion, spirituality, and health: New considerations for epidemiology. *American Journal of Epidemiology, 189*(8), 755–758.

Raudon, N. (2023). *Huddled masses: Death and citizenship in New York City* (Doctoral dissertation, Cambridge University, Cambridge, England).

Restorative Justice. (2023, November). *LISTENING TO SURVIVORS OF GUN VIOLENCE THROUGH A RESTORATIVE JUSTICE LENS: THE PRESCRIPTIONS FOR REPAIR PROJECT Final Report.* https://nonviolentdurham.org/wp-content/uploads/P4R-Final-Report.pdf

Rice, H. E., Owen, M., Johnson, A., Swandell, J., Nicholson, C. P., Provencher, S., et al. (2024). Lived experiences of people impacted by gun violence: Qualitative analysis of the prescriptions for repair project. *Trauma Surgery & Acute Care Open, 9*(1), e001503.

Ross, K. M., Sullivan, T., O'Connor, K., Hitti, S., & Leiva, M. N. (2021). A community-specific framework of risk factors for youth violence: A qualitative comparison of community stakeholder perspectives in a low-income, urban community. *Journal of Community Psychology, 49*(5), 1134–1152.

Ross, K. M., Walsh, C. S., Angulo, A. G., Leslie, C. E., & Tolan, P. H. (2024). Evidence-based strategies for preventing urban youth violence. In D. P. Mears (Ed.), *The Oxford handbook of evidence-based crime and justice policy* (pp. 444–465). Oxford University Press.

Rynearson, E. K., & Salloum, A. (2021). Restoratuve Retelling: Revising the narrative of violent death. In R. A. Neimeyer, D. L. Harris, H. R. Winokver & G. Thorton. (Eds.). *Grief and Bereavement in Contemporary Society*. Routledge Publishers.

Sandberg, B., Hurmerinta, L., & Menzfeld, M. (2024). Volunteerism and community healing. *Community Development, 55*(6), 795-801-15.

Schladen, M. (2024, February 20). Human, financial costs of gun violence are growing dramatically, health care group says. *Ohio Capital Journal.* https://ohiocapitaljournal.com/2024/02/20/human-financial-costs-of-gun-violence-are-growing-dramatically-health-care-group-says/

Stager, C. G., Whitfield, S., Osborne, T., Adedoyin, C., Okoro, G., Carley, E., et al. (2024). Community perceptions of contributors and solutions related to neighborhood violent crime: A qualitative interview study. *Journal of Community Psychology, 52*(2), 311–325.

Walker, I. A., Smith Lee, J. R., Payton Foh, E., McKoy, P., & Johnson, M. H. (2024). "Resilience looks like me": Community stakeholder perspectives on resilience in Black boys and young men exposed to community violence. *American Psychologist, 79*(8), 1092.

Weisburd, D., Groff, E. R., & Yang, S. M. (2012). *The criminology of place: Street segments and our understanding of the crime problem.* Oxford University Press.

Windle, T. (2024). *Tailored therapeutic musical theater community engagement project.* Leslie University. https://digitalcommons.lesley.edu/cgi/viewcontent.cgi?article=1785&context=expressive_theses

Index

© The Editor(s) (if applicable) and The Author(s), under exclusive license to Springer Nature Switzerland AG 2025
M. Delgado, *The Death Care Industry and Urban Gun Violence*,
https://doi.org/10.1007/978-3-031-95682-9

GPSR Compliance
The European Union's (EU) General Product Safety Regulation (GPSR) is a set of rules that requires consumer products to be safe and our obligations to ensure this.

If you have any concerns about our products, you can contact us on

ProductSafety@springernature.com

In case Publisher is established outside the EU, the EU authorized representative is:

Springer Nature Customer Service Center GmbH
Europaplatz 3
69115 Heidelberg, Germany

v.ingramcontent.com/pod-product-compliance
ning Source LLC
ersburg PA
51031140725
300001B/11
7 8 3 0 3 1 9 5 6 8 1 2 *